Lupus
My Search
for a Diagnosis

EILEEN RADZIUNAS holds a bachelor's degree in education and has taught public school at the elementary level. Prior to her illness she was active as a volunteer in her community schools. Since being diagnosed as having lupus, she founded and runs a lupus support group in her area and is extremely active in lupus education.

She feels her most important qualification for writing this book is the painful experience of having an "imposter disease," and working with others in the same situation. She wishes to increase public knowledge about imposter diseases and, through this book and other means of education, to speed the search for a cure.

Eileen Radziunas lives with her husband and daughters in Higganum, Connecticut.

Kathleen West has a Masters in Public Health and lives in Los Angeles, where she works as a Program Development Director for programs affiliated with the King/Drew Medical Center in Watts. She has a background in medical anthropology and maternal and child health, and has done most of her work in "cross-cultural" health care settings. She considers the world of medicine to be one of the most challenging "cultures" with which people are called upon to interface. Her older sister has spent more than fifteen years searching for a definitive diagnosis of her disease.

To Eddie, Stacey, and Storey,
my three best incentives
for fighting this illness.

With special thanks to the rheumatologist I now see,
for believing me from the day I first walked into his office
and, in so doing, immeasurably improving
the quality of my life.

Lupus

My Search for a Diagnosis

by

E<small>ILEEN</small> R<small>ADZIUNAS</small>

Edited by Jackie Melvin

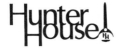

Library of Congress Cataloging in Publication Data:
Radziunas, Eileen
Lupus: my search for a diagnosis / Eileen Radziunas:
edited by Jackie Melvin.—1st U.S. ed.
p.   cm.
ISBN 0-89793-065-7 : $6.95
1. Radziunas, Eileen—Health. 2. Systemic lupus
erythematosus—Patients—United States—Biography.
3. Systemic lupus erythematosus—Diagnosis.
I. Melvin, Jackie. II. Title.
RC924.5.L85R33   1989
616.7'7—dc20   89-24683

Book and cover design by Qalagraphia
Cover illustration by Renee Krikken
Production manager: Paul J. Frindt
Set in 10½ on 13 point Bookman
by 847 Communications, Claremont, CA
Printed and bound by Patterson Printing, Benton Harbor, MI
Manufactured in the United States of America

9 8 7 6 5 4 3 2   First edition

Contents

Doctor's Foreword
by Kevin Michaels, M.D.

I have followed Eileen Radziunas since 1984, through her diagnosis of a connective tissue disease. When I first read *Lupus: My Search for a Diagnosis,* my heart went out even further to Eileen for the effort she made to prove to the medical profession that she was really ill. I began examining my conscience about how little physicians really understand about patients' true feelings. While not a day goes by without some new technological advance, we doctors must constantly remember that we are not omnipotent.

Eileen was more than willing at times to accept the statement, "I just don't know, but I believe you and what you are saying." She reiterates this many times through the book: she just wanted to be believed.

Through the years I have gotten to know Eileen, not only as a patient but as a friend. As difficult as it is to come up with a diagnosis, she kept fighting through thick and thin. While her emotional support may not have come through the medical profession, her family certainly provided it. I realize that the uniqueness of Eileen is in part a result of a very strong family. I was delighted that Eileen wrote this book. She continues to struggle and hopefully will be able to relieve her pain. I feel her book ought to be required reading for anyone in the medical field, and anyone with a chronic illness. She has certainly changed my life, and my understanding of myself.

Foreword

by Kathleen M. West, M.P.H.

Eileen Radziunas's moving story will certainly influence me in my professional work in the areas of public health, health care advocacy, and physician-patient communication. It has certainly deepened my commitment to help bridge the communication gap that all too often exists between patients and doctors. But I must confess that the real reason for my avid reading of her story is the fact that my older sister is *still* searching for that elusive definitive diagnosis of lupus, more than fifteen years after her initial symptoms appeared. The diagnosis of "collagen-vascular disease of unknown etiology" with "suspected" lupus erythematosus is the closest my sister has come to a formal diagnosis.

As a result, my introductory words here are directed primarily toward the family members and friends of people who have or think they may have lupus, as well as to health care providers and patient advocates. Many of you in the first category, of family, may also find yourselves in the second category, since so many of us as family members gradually learn how to be patient advocates and "lay" case managers for our loved ones.

I only need to focus for a moment to remember my sister's ailments, or look in my top desk drawer in the file entitled: "Sharon's Health Status" to keep myself up-to-date with her long list of medical diagnoses. These include: adult onset diabetes, hyperlipidemia, temporomandibular joint syndrome, multiple granulomas, several experiences of anaphylactic shock, Raynaud's phenomenon, swelling of the joints, bronchitis, proteinuria, systemic candidiasis, pericarditis, mouth ulcers, sinusitis, and multiple ongoing problems involving the pulmonary, reproductive, renal, and immunologic systems. Sharon's medical records must rival the Los Angeles and New York phone books in volume! Because I am involved in the health care field, the above list of diseases and disease processes conveys some meaning to me of how very sick my sister is. But as a generally healthy person, who grew up knowing my sister to *also* be a healthy person, I cannot truly imagine what it is like to suffer those diseases as my daily existence.

As a health care worker, I was taught primarily how to help people arrive at a desired *outcome* when they entered the health care system. The desired outcome that Western medicine usually aims at is a cure, or "health." While this goal is inarguably a good one in most cases, it has caused us to overlook the *process* whereby we give and receive health care. The poor treatment Eileen describes receiving at the hands of the medical profession provided her with neither a cure nor peace of mind. She arrived at the latter largely through use of her own resources, *despite* the medical system. Because we do not yet have answers or "cures" for a large number of devastating and sometimes hard-to-diagnose diseases, like lupus, those of us in the health care field *must* learn to maximize what we *do* have: patients who can reliably tell us what is happening to them, and our own compassion and empathy to advocate for them as best we can within an often foreign and complicated system.

Eileen's generous sharing of her story helped me to have some insight into the reality of being a for-

eigner in the health care world and gave me an opportunity to step into the subculture of those living in
constant pain, dis-ease, and perhaps as bad or
worse, nagging self-doubt and fear that one will not
be taken seriously. The burden of constantly having
to legitimize oneself to the medical establishment is
recounted by Eileen and *felt* by the reader to be *exhausting.*

While I never dismissed my sister's symptoms
and feelings of ill health, I am sorry to say that, as a
family member, at times I became so exasperated and
perplexed at the uncertainty of my sister's medical
condition that all I displayed was downright anger
and impatience. We in the Western world are *so* uncomfortable with unanswered questions that we want
to deny the *reality* of anything we don't have answers
to! I certainly wanted to deny my sister's incapacity
to join in family activities, to feel well for a sustained
period of time, and to GET BETTER. "Magical thinking" is not limited to children!

As a young adult with the world ahead of me, in
a society that worships health and fitness, I saw my
sister's "weird" illnesses as an affront of sorts. Her
easy fatigue was offensive to my high energy level.
Though in my heart of hearts I usually felt compassion, sympathy, and supportiveness, I did not always
express that to her. Fortunately, most of the time my
sister was able to read between the lines and interpreted my anger and disappointment as the fear and
sense of helplessness that it really was.

As I read *Lupus: My Search for a Diagnosis*, I was
impressed, therefore, with Eileen's faithful circle of
family and friends. Having experienced chronic debilitating diseases both in my work and my family, I
know that Eileen's fortunate experience with supportive family and friends is far from universal. Much

more common are the harsh self-judgments, internal arguments, and bewilderment that Eileen describes, as doctor after doctor can find "no basis in fact" for painful symptoms, and friend after friend becomes less sympathetic as one's illness continues to go unnamed.

As a family member of one who has lupus (definitively diagnosed or not!), I would urge other family members to do the following five things:

1. *Read this book*, but don't stop at that;

2. Take Eileen's story to heart, *and* take her story to your ill family member or friend. Ask them if/how it "rings true" in their experience or how their experience differs. Giving your sick, tired, and worried family member or friend a chance to talk about their problems may be the most helpful thing you can do;

3. Don't assume that listening is the *only* thing you can do. Ask if there are ways you can help, and then listen to the meaning and tone behind the words and listen for unspoken words. If, like Eileen, your family member or friend is having a difficult time coordinating their medical care, you can help. And you don't have to be a health professional to do it. You just have to *not* be intimidated by the medical profession, and you have to use "forceful diplomacy." I have found that the common missing link in all the complicated cases with which I have worked is case management. While this is something that one primary physician *should* do, you can help to ensure that it happens

by pulling together all the disparate medical records, test results, doctor's names, etc. into one place. Several years ago, I did just that with my sister. We reconstructed the last ten years of *her* search for a diagnosis, composed a three-page letter, and sent it to her primary doctor with copies to eleven other physicians. Within weeks, her medical records began to come together and better resolution of her case has happened since.

4. Learn all you can about the possible disease and disease processes, talk with your friend or family member to hear what particular questions/problems they're having, and then accompany them to a doctor's appointment and politely but firmly ask questions. (And, take what is said with a grain of salt. Remember, the medical profession is not God, and is still in the learning process itself— especially about diseases that involve an interplay of different organ systems and the immune system.) In this way, you can serve as a patient advocate, and save your loved one a lot of extra effort. Last, but not least,

5. Encourage your family member or friend to get involved in a local support or self-help group—and get involved yourself. Hearing the stories and strategies for coping, as well as learning of new resources that others have, is both inspirational and helpful. These groups have a hard time functioning at an optimal level without *some* support from able-bodied friends and family, so make yourself available!

Preface

Living with lupus is one of the most difficult challenges I have ever had to face. It is a frightening, unpredictable disease which seems to reveal new symptoms every day. I often feel as though I am sitting on a keg of dynamite, never knowing when a major organ will be attacked and I will need immediate hospitalization. Beyond a doubt, it is a disease which demands continual professional supervision and effective doctor/patient communication.

Although the physical disabilities associated with lupus can be overwhelming, the lingering emotional scars from my long search for a diagnosis are far more devastating, and perhaps irreparable. The humiliation and self-doubt I felt from not being believed— for such a long time, by so many key people—have been shattering to my self-confidence. This loss of trust has actually been the most destructive element of the illness. I felt ignored and pacified by condescending physicians who undermined my intelligence and questioned my sanity. They were obviously in a far better position than I to call the shots, and influenced each other repeatedly in the way my case was handled. My anger built daily as I was forced to battle extreme pain on my own. I now know that much of that pain could have been treated, if I had been believed earlier.

Though I find some consolation in the fact that I also saw many dedicated, caring physicians, I attribute my successful management of this illness and an immeasurably improved quality of life to finding a physician who consistently respected and believed what I had to say—which is no more than any patient deserves. By working with me, rather than in spite of me, he was able to diagnose and begin to treat my disease.

I try to remain hopeful that my case will go into remission, as this is a disease which can become more disabling the further it progresses. I know that other people with serious cases have gone from severe disability to being able to work again. I am also encouraged that these "imposter diseases" are being more extensively researched, and remain optimistic that a more effective treatment will be discovered—or even better, a cure.

I wrote this book to increase our general awareness and understanding of lupus, so that this mysterious disease can begin to be diagnosed earlier. I hope that sharing the intimacies of my experience will show that a serious disease process can be taking place long before clinically significant test results appear. This applies not only to lupus, but to other "imposter diseases" as well, such as multiple sclerosis, Epstein-Barr virus, endometriosis, and temporomandibular joint syndrome (some of these are discussed in Appendix II).

I want to give chronically ill patients the message that there is hope. You have little control over the fact that you have a certain disease, but you can control the way you respond to it, and that can strongly influence your ability to cope and to heal. You do have choices.

Speaking from difficult experience, I know that it isn't easy. But I also know that there is much you can do to help yourself. Get more than one medical opinion, if you are not satisfied. Educate yourself about possible diagnoses. Many people grow through counseling or support groups. Try visualization, prayer, relaxation tapes, gentle exercise. Maintaining warm and honest relations with your family and friends is, of course, central to your physical and emotional health.

My most important message to you is: *Don't give up.* Living with a chronic illness is a daily struggle, but your inner resources are powerful tools and can truly make a difference.

While many people did not believe me during that first year, I managed, with the support of a few very special people, to continue to believe in myself. I hope that my story will help patients—and doctors—recognize that we can avoid a great deal of needless pain through our ongoing efforts to make our lives as whole and healthy as possible.

Prologue

If, on the eve of the new year, 1984, someone could have told me about the drastic change that was about to occur in my life, I never would have celebrated. Perhaps it is lucky that no one had that power of prediction.

My husband, Eddie, and I drove off, as we had for several years, to our town dance, looking forward to enjoying another New Year's Eve with our closest friends. The party was well under way when we arrived, and our friends hailed us from a table near the dance floor.

The evening was full of lively, comfortable conversation and the kind of friendly teasing that only takes place with very good friends. We recalled humorous events from past New Year's parties, and sought out other friends in the crowd. What I remember most about the evening is that we danced to the point of exhaustion, with each "golden oldie" reviving memories for us all.

As midnight approached, we put on festive hats, blew on our noisemakers, poured more champagne and headed again for the dance floor. Balloons cascaded from the ceiling as the clock struck twelve; a New Year's baby ran through the crowd. We kissed our partners and wished everyone a wonderful year to come.

It was the perfect start to a new year: talking about the past, sharing the moment, and making resolutions for the future. Or so it seemed at the time. I did not realize that my life was about to change completely. This is my story.

1

The Accident

It was a brisk January evening in 1984. A stinging, invigorating chill hit my cheeks as I walked toward the health club. I was there to introduce my new friend Carrie to racquetball. I was looking forward to sharing some common involvement with Carrie, whose enthusiasm seemed to have no bounds.

She turned out to be a natural on the court. Within half an hour she was familiar with the rules and comfortable with the game. Early on, while I was demonstrating a forehand shot, I overextended my arm and felt the zing of what I guessed was a pulled muscle in my lower back. I had to cut back a great deal, but, unwilling to call this first session short, I convinced myself that I could handle a few more minutes. I didn't mention the pain to Carrie.

When I got up for work the next day, the discomfort from the "pulled muscle" had intensified. I was working as a receptionist in the office of a physician, Dr. Dupont, who was also my own doctor, and though I was reminded of the pain several times that day, I decided not to mention my injury to him. I had an unfortunate and painful experience with doctors early in my life, and I have never been fond of examinations. I hoped this pain was something minor which would go away on its own.

After four or five days had passed, with the pain intensifying, it became unnervingly clear that this was *not* a minor injury. The pain wasn't intolerable, but it began to interrupt my sleep. I tried to concentrate on other things—Eddie and I were about to leave on our annual weekend away, and I was caught up in our daughters' enthusiasm for their weekend with their grandfather. Stacey and Storey kept me busy as I tried to put the pain out of my mind. We live in a small town in Connecticut, and this year Eddie and I had decided to stay at a Vermont ski resort. Though neither of us are skiers, the resort offered so many other amenities that we wanted to investigate it as a timesharing possibility.

Although I worried to myself about the extent of this injury, I had been anticipating the weekend for so long that I stubbornly refused to forfeit it. Eddie needed a vacation too; his work as a systems consultant was demanding, and he'd put in many long hours since we'd last had any relaxing time together.

As we headed north, we ran into freezing rain, which extended the three-hour trip by another painful hour. My back and legs were extremely uncomfortable, no matter how I positioned myself.

By the time we arrived at the resort, I needed help getting out of the car. My spirits were dampened, but I chose to believe that things would improve now that the drive was over. We had a lovely late night meal together, and discussed our weekend plans over a bottle of wine.

Since we had arrived after dark, the scene from the picture window in the lodge the next morning was especially breathtaking. Sunbathed, snow-covered mountains surrounded us. The only distraction from the great beauty around us was my increasing pain. I could only walk for short periods, and had to favor my right leg throughout the morning. We tried to explore the grounds, but I could barely put any weight on that leg, and finally I was forced to go back to our room to lie down.

Surprisingly, the pain only became worse during the afternoon as I rested. I fought back tears—this was not the vacation I'd been looking forward to! I tried to convince Eddie to go to dinner without me, but he stayed, leaving only to call the girls to say goodnight.

At breakfast the next morning, we talked candidly. The scenery was terrific and it was wonderful to be alone, but my pain was just incredible. The only logical thing to do was leave and promise ourselves another weekend away as soon as I was better.

Dr. Dupont noticed that I was favoring my right leg when I went back to work on Monday. I finally admitted to him that I had pain traveling down my leg. He recommended an exam to rule out a disk injury, and although I was unenthusiastic about the suggestion, his serious tone told me that he felt the exam was essential. This would be the first of countless exams for me—a year of them before I would discover what was wrong.

His exam did not reveal any sign of a disk injury. My ankle jerk reflexes were normal, which he found encouraging, and I had considerable mobility—much more than most patients with disk problems. I was relieved to think that whatever I had was not serious; probably some type of inflammation, which Dr. Dupont felt might respond to muscle relaxants.

Eddie was scheduled to chair the annual Wives' Appreciation Dinner the next night for the local Jaycees.

I always look forward to these evenings, but this was one of the most difficult social functions I have ever had to attend. We drove out of town with several close friends and, while it was only twenty minutes to the restaurant, the intensity of my pain during that brief ride is unforgettable. I was burning from my knees to my thighs. I couldn't keep up with the conversation at all, unable to concentrate on anything but the pain.

Socializing became even more difficult at the restaurant. Surrounded by this large, less familiar group of people, I simply could not respond to anyone. Just sitting there was difficult. I tried to hide my discomfort, but a good friend sitting next to me could see what was happening. Both she and Eddie suggested leaving early, but I felt that Eddie should remain through the evening, since he was the chair. And I didn't want to curtail my friends' evening by making them leave with me. In retrospect, it was a foolish decision. There were other people who could have taken over for Eddie, and our friends would have found rides home with someone else. I stayed, stubbornly. I fought back tears as the evening went on, and all the way home.

The pain deep in my thighs was more intense as I sat at work the next day. The muscle relaxants had not helped at all. My legs felt so heavy, as though I couldn't lift them. (As it turns out, the word "heavy" was an unfortunate choice on my part, because many doctors associate it with psychosomatic complaints.)

My physician suggested a chiropractor, and I immediately refused. I was a definite skeptic about chiropractic medicine. Eddie had been urging me to see one, and now my doctor had jumped on the bandwagon. Considering my intense discomfort, however, and out of sheer desperation, I finally made an appointment.

I had not expected the variety of equipment and array of treatments that the chiropractor had to offer. He took an X-ray of my back, which revealed no disk involvement, but which did show that my back was out of alignment. The chiropractor applied electrical charges to my back and manipulated my spine. It was a weird sensation, though nothing hurt. I left in as much pain as when I arrived. Eddie encouraged me to withhold judgment until I'd given the treatment a chance.

When I returned the following week, I was assigned to the senior partner in the group, who informed me that the problem was not in my back but my knees, based on the sensitivity I showed when he examined them. The idea sounded incredible to me, given my severe back pain, but I had to admit that I also had significant discomfort in my right knee. The chiropractor prescribed a series of daily exercises. This struck me as ludicrous—I was barely able to move. I left the office frustrated, and in more pain than ever. I called Dr. Dupont to report my condition, and let him know that I had no intention of returning to the chiropractor. He and Eddie tried to convince me to change my mind, but the decision was mine.

The lower back and leg pain increased, getting in the way of my everyday activities—driving in the carpool, cooking, volunteering at school, socializing. I had to take my first sick leave, and Dr. Dupont restricted me to complete bedrest for five days. Though I strictly followed his advice, the pain continued. Pain medication did not help me sleep through the night. I had a burning pain in my legs, and a "pins and needles" sensation developed on the soles of my feet.

At the end of my bedrest and in consultation with my doctor, I was sent to a neurosurgeon to check once again on the possibility of disk disease. When I needed Eddie to drive me the half-hour distance, I began to realize that this injury was more serious than I'd been willing to believe. I had always equated neurosurgery with frightening medical problems, such as brain tumors. My doctor relieved some of my fears, letting me know that neurosurgeons are often recommended for back surgery because of the delicate nature of the operation.

This meeting turned out to be a positive one. The surgeon was easy to communicate with. I had lost my right ankle reflex since the last exam. This development, and my description of the pain, made him suspect a ruptured disk. Verifying that would require admission to the hospital and a CAT scan.

I can't say we were surprised. It was no news to us that something was very wrong. But Eddie and I were caught off guard by the doctor's insistence that I go in the very next day. His urgency was generated by the location of the disk he guessed was involved; disk trouble in the lumbar region—the lower back—carries the threat of serious complications, including the loss of bowel and bladder control. I was determined to avoid any more trouble, and agreed to be admitted the next day on the surgeon's assurance that he would not consider surgery unless it was absolutely necessary.

At the hospital that next day, the surgeon explained that the CAT scan was the first step in a process. If the scan did not definitively identify the problem, a myelogram would be needed. I had heard horror stories about this procedure, in which a long needle is inserted into the spine, and I cringed at the suggestion.

Before the CAT scan was administered, I asked the technician if there was anything I could do to lessen the chance that I would need a myelogram. She said that I should lie as still as possible during the scan, so that the picture would be very clear. I could have been a statue. The technician could not give me any results immediately, but I left the room feeling confident that the surgeon would be satisfied with the scan findings.

I learned during afternoon rounds that I would hear nothing about the scan until the next day, so I accepted the prescribed sleeping pill and pain medication and let my body drift into a long sleep.

The next morning the surgeon described to me a large ruptured disk revealed by the CAT scan. I was concerned, but not surprised. In fact, I was relieved; this meant I wouldn't need a myelogram. A few minutes later, however, the surgeon let me know that he also wanted a myelogram done to clarify the extent of the injury. I asked a hundred questions about the procedure, which I'd heard was so painful. The surgeon answered each of my questions thoroughly, and then administered the exam skillfully, explaining each step. Though the procedure was not painless, most of my fears proved to be a combination of a very normal fear of the unknown and exaggerated stories I'd heard which I would have been better off ignoring.

I now knew that my fifth lumbar disk had ruptured, with damage on both sides. This was almost certainly the cause of the pain that was now shooting down both legs. I had managed to avoid the dreadful headache I had heard follows a myelogram, and went to sleep knowing that I would need surgery. Just before I fell asleep, I noticed that my arms were burning—a sensation identical to that in my legs. I tried to remind myself to tell the surgeon about this in the morning.

Eddie and I had some difficulty making the decision to go ahead with the back surgery. A friend whose medical advice my husband had always trusted spoke out against back surgery and emphasized the risks involved. Eddie was visibly nervous and pressured me to avoid surgery, fearing that the end result might be crippling. He was so alarmed that we consulted two other physicians. They reassured us: It was successive surgeries, rather than the initial operation, that caused most back complications. They convinced us further by letting us know that surgery would be their personal choice if they had the same problem.

So, why, with all this good advice, did I hesitate during the discussion that next morning with Eddie and the surgeon? It was that burning sensation throughout my body, the tingling which by now was in my feet and hands. It was painful to have a blood pressure cuff wrapped around my arm, and more painful when it was pumped up. I didn't see how these sensations could be related to the ruptured disk, and I was scared. I needed to talk about these developments now, before the surgery.

I initiated a conversation about my symptoms, but the surgeon responded by telling me that he could not explain them. He *was* sure that a disk injury in the lower lumbar area could not be responsible for the arm sensations I described. This particular combination of symptoms "did not make medical sense." Perhaps I was simply anxious about having surgery? I disputed the inference that I was concocting my symptoms; I had had surgery before and knew something about what to expect.

In a final effort to allay my fears and at the same

time confirm his diagnosis, the surgeon requested my permission for a neurological consult. The doctor he had in mind was very knowledgeable about peripheral nerve involvement, which I seemed to be describing. My surgeon felt sure that this man would recognize any neurological problem that might exist.

The neurologist seemed dedicated enough when he appeared, but I was less impressed with him than my surgeon had been. Perhaps it was the nature of the exam that bothered me, or the implications of what he might find. The patient with whom I shared a room had been diagnosed with a brain tumor, and I had seen firsthand how her family reacted to the news. The woman was frightened and shared her feelings openly with me. I had heard her physician present the news in a cold, tactless way.

As the neurologist asked me to close my eyes and bring my finger to my nose, to feel for pinpricks, and to follow a light, I feared that I might be about to receive the same frightening news. Instead, he also suggested that I was just anxious about the upcoming surgery, and recommended that I go ahead with it. He also commented that I had been nervous during the exam. Of course I was nervous! Considering the types of illness he might have discovered, I felt my nervousness was justifiable and I told him so.

My thoughts that evening focused on my doubts about everything that was about to happen to me. I fought with the corners of the fitted sheets, and felt intruded upon by the constant paging over the intercom. I was not at all certain that this surgery was the best choice.

What a relief to see Sue and Jen, two of my closest friends, walk in just then, red-cheeked and shivering from the cold night air. We'd been friends for about ten years. Low-key, easygoing Sue is one of the best listeners I know, never failing to consider all sides of a situation, which makes her advice all the more valuable. Reliable and patient, she seems to anticipate other people's needs. Jen is the most direct and unique of my friends. I frequently ask her opinion and count on her for an honest answer. Her dry sense of humor never fails to make me laugh.

None of us laughed that night, unfortunately, as I shared my growing doubts about the next day. It was an intense visit. As Sue and Jen got up to leave, I shared my deepest fear—that this pain was not going to end with tomorrow's surgery.

Late that night my worried thoughts were interrupted by a call from Dr. Dupont. I updated him on my latest symptoms, including the new sensations in my arms, which he found puzzling. I bombarded him with questions for which he, also, had no answers.

All I could do was try to sleep, though I was frustrated, and profoundly apprehensive.

2

Back Surgery—
and More

Early the next morning, as I signed a "Consent for Surgery" form, the surgeon and I chatted blithely about having nothing better to do on this dreary, rainy day. He commented, in a questioning tone, as if thinking out loud, on the surprising amount of mobility I had for someone with such severe disk damage. I have wondered since if this mobility might not have been an important, overlooked clue that the ruptured disk was not responsible for the pain I was experiencing.

The surgeon took down Eddie's phone number for a post-op call, and I was pre-medicated and wheeled to the surgical area. I distinctly remember the surgeon saying that whatever was happening with my arms could not possibly be corrected by this back surgery. But as I lay there, the feelings in my arms were identical to those in my legs. How could I be sure my leg pains would improve? Was surgery the wrong answer? I began to shake uncontrollably as the anesthetic was administered. Later, my surgeon told me that I had vigorously fought going to sleep. I'm sure that my doubts about the operation were responsible.

Although at one point during the surgery my blood pressure dropped dangerously low, everything else proceeded normally, and I was only in the recovery room a short time. It was such a relief to be back in my bed, with Eddie sitting beside me. The pain in my arms and legs was gone! Now I felt that we'd made the right choice. The surgeon stopped by to let me know that the ruptured disk had been very large. He was pleased, under the circumstances, to see me so cheerful.

Eddie had brought a bouquet of yellow roses. He was wearing the biggest smile I had seen on him in weeks, because I felt so positive about the surgery. As he left the room to return home, the phone rang. It was Jen, in a "too afraid to ask" voice, checking up on me. I had come to depend on and anticipate her daily calls, and this one was especially good, because I had a chance to share my euphoria over this remarkable lack of pain. When she was finally able to get a word in, Jen just sighed with relief. We promised to talk again the next day.

My elation proved premature; I had not taken into account the benefits of the anesthesia. As it began to wear off, the pain returned. The site of my incision was now far less painful than my arms and legs! What now? I tried to make it clear to the nurses who administered my pain medication that I needed it for my entire body, and not specifically for the new incision. I wasn't holding back the tears anymore. I just cried—from discouragement, frustration, and fear.

The surgeon and I talked repeatedly. He was perplexed by my complaints. He began to inquire about my home life, my children, work. I answered his questions as honestly as I could. . . . I was not upset, I was *sick*. In his opinion, my symptoms simply did not add up to any known illness.

New problems appeared later in the week of my hospital stay. My lips and tongue became numb. My left hand became completely numb from the wrist to the tips of my fingers. The surgeon consulted with Dr. Dupont and ordered more blood tests. Every test came back "normal."

Because my surgeon was off the following weekend, his associate made rounds. It was the first time we'd met, and I immediately felt uncomfortable with him. He rushed into the room, giving the distinct impression that he would rather be anywhere else. I began to feel fortunate that I'd been referred to his partner, and found myself wondering how two such opposites could have a successful practice together. He made a point of letting me know that I looked like I was doing "just fine." I quickly informed him that I was *not* fine. I was experiencing more of the pins and needles numbness than ever. The burning pain in my extremities had not subsided at all. It hurt now just to rest my arms against the sheets.

After listening for a few minutes, the doctor left to find a pin. He tested for sensation in several areas and summarily informed me that not one of my complaints was neurological in nature. He was convinced that I had a deep-rooted psychological problem which was responsible for the pain. He suggested that I "do something about it" immediately, and left the room.

I began to understand what had happened. He had read my chart, which by now contained several notations to the effect that my symptoms did not make "good medical sense." I realized that my treatment had changed considerably in the last few days, and that this doctor's blunt commentary was merely part of an overall change in attitude toward me. The doctor had begun to ask me why I didn't watch television. I was criticized for this, and told that it was a sign of depression. I am not a TV fan; I am a reader. The fact that I read several novels during my stay did not seem to count.

The nursing staff also had access to my chart, of course. As I put the pieces together, I recalled that whenever I mentioned the now very severe pain to the nurses, it was downplayed. I began to see that I was in a no-win situation, and my fear began to change to anger.

I woke up on Sunday morning to the unnerving realization that my sheets were not clammy from the stifling temperature in the hospital, but because I had lost control of my bladder in my sleep. I panicked. I shook myself awake, and struggled to regain control of my body. I started to sweat and cry and tremble.

Every moment seemed incredibly long. It took many rings of the bedside buzzer before a frazzled nurse appeared. She recorded this latest development with an undisguised look of surprise.

My worst fear was that this could be related to multiple sclerosis. Though I knew very little about that disease, I remembered a conversation with a friend, years earlier, about a relative who had MS. What I recalled about that talk was that incontinence was one of the symptoms of MS, and that eventually this woman had been confined to a wheelchair.

As I lay there, with pain throughout my muscles, my mind was racing. The possibility that this might be a terribly serious disease depressed me. I wished that I had access to a book on MS at that very moment, so I could determine whether my fears had any basis.

The nurse interrupted my thoughts with the suggestion that I "lie back and relax." Relax! How dare she expect me to relax when terrifying changes were happening to my body, with no explanation? I wondered how relaxed she or my doctors would be if they had just experienced such a moment: waking up to discover another serious complication, more frightening loss of control.

I needed to talk to Eddie. I needed to tell my fears to someone I knew would understand. His support had been constant throughout this illness. Maybe because our relationship began as good friends, living near each other in a small town, after 13 years of marriage we had the ability to communicate with each other as only close friends do. If I ever needed him, it was now.

The telephone was in the hall. I leaned against the phone for support and shook as I dialed our number. Buzzers rang, trays slammed, the intercom screeched, and a dozen conversations went on around me. When Eddie answered, I burst into tears just hearing his voice. I tried to describe the incontinence and the lack of compassion from the doctor and staff.

Eddie's voice was subdued, and I knew it was from fear or nervousness. What was happening to me was also painful for him. He had witnessed my daily physical changes and increasing pain, and had his own doubts and frustrations about the hospital and the surgery. My health had become the focus of all our conversations. Looking back, there must have been more creative options for us, but all I can remember is that we felt defeated. I was exhausted physically and mentally, and Eddie had an extended workload between his job and caring for the girls in my absence. We were both concerned about alarming the girls, which was another burden. Eddie promised to come as quickly as he could, and to bring Stacey and Storey.

I took a shower in preparation for their visit, which meant I had to go down the hall again. My legs felt weighted down, as though someone were pulling them into the floor. In the shower, I reached for the handrail, and fell against it like a dead weight. When I had showered and regained a little strength, I dressed, walked out into the antiseptic corridor and, using the smooth oak rails along the walls for support, made it back to my room. I had to lean against the wall several times to get to my bed on the far side of the room.

The cold metal siderail felt good against my burning skin. I was relieved, for the moment, that the incontinence had stopped, but concerned as to what it meant. Stacey had loaned me her canary yellow transistor radio, and I picked it up, trying to find some music which might help me get a little rest.

As I waited, I overheard a conversation across the hall. The woman in that room was also in her thirties, and had been admitted for the same type of surgery on the same day that I was. She was arranging for transportation, about to be discharged. I had spoken to her several times, and she had let me know quite clearly that she did not believe we were suffering from the same problem. Her worst discomfort had been from the back incision, and she had never experienced the numbness, burning, or muscle pain which I continued to feel. Each day she grew stronger and able to do more, while I grew worse. I had had abdominal surgery years before, and recovered quickly. Wishing that were the case now, I felt depressed listening to her excited voice.

Lost in my thoughts, I heard her enter my room. She was carrying one of her prettiest flower arrangements, and gave me a hug, saying that she hoped the flowers would bring me luck. I know she was trying to help, but her reassurance that the doctors would "get to the bottom of all this soon" was less than convincing. My eyes filled with tears as she left.

Within minutes, Eddie and the girls walked into the room. Afraid that the girls would see my discouragement, I blinked my eyes dry and struggled to make an effort to smile. Apparently I was convincing, because each of them ran over with a kiss and a hug, not questioning the transparency of my emotions. Eddie's eyes, however, were knowing; I had not fooled him.

We had agreed that the first part of the visit needed to be dedicated to the girls, but I found it hard to let Eddie go. I wanted to cry in his arms, let him hold me, but I told myself that we would have that time alone later.

I had not seen Stacey and Storey for five days, and based on the apprehension I sensed in our phone calls, I knew that being together now was very important. *I* needed uninterrupted time with each of them as much as they needed me. Throughout this illness, I had been preoccupied with my family. However serious this problem was for me, it also weighed heavily on each of the people I loved.

Storey and Stacey experimented with the automatic bed until I was practically dizzy, and argued over who would get the fluffy stuffed animal my brothers had sent. How young my girls were! Stacey was eight and Storey just four, and I knew they were perhaps more dependent on me than they needed to be. From their early infancy, we took part in play groups, swim lessons, and gymnastics. We went to the weekly story hour at the library, and had memorable birthday parties with hayrides, sleep-overs, scavenger hunts, and face-painting clowns. Being their mother was rewarding, challenging, and essential. Never before had I considered that all this could change, but here it was, our life completely altered before my disbelieving eyes.

As I watched my girls play, the thought entered my mind for the first time since my injury that I might have a fatal disease. I know now that this was the direct result of having no name for the frightening physical changes overtaking my body. Praying to God that I was wrong, I asked myself whether I could actually be fatally ill without any medical detection, after so many tests. I could not deny the validity of my pain. Maybe the doctors were not making any connections at this point, but I was.

Suddenly it became imperative for me to be wrong. It was a great disservice to Eddie, but I was convinced that no one could raise my children like I could, or understand their needs. I wanted to be wrong about this new fear, but some inner feeling haunted me: I might be closer to the mark than all of the professionals and their technology. My daughters never looked more precious.

Storey helped herself to a handful of my chocolates—a treat that was rarely permitted at home—and headed off down the hall with Eddie. I wrapped my arm around Stacey, who was stretched out next to me in bed. As happy as I was to be with her, I had to wince from the pain of her weight against my skin.

She seemed taller than I remembered. I ached with helplessness listening to her describe how much she missed me and how worried she was. Her freshly washed hair smelled sweet and familiar. I could tell by the fluctuations in her voice and by her concerted effort to maintain a brave appearance that she had guessed the truth—the surgery had not cured me as we had hoped. She asked more and more questions. I tried to be as reassuring as I could, but with my own monumental doubts, I knew I was not completely believable. Though our time together was special, it was unsettling, I think, for both of us.

Stacey left, and Storey came back in, climbing up onto the bed with yet another handful of chocolate! How could I refuse those impish brown eyes? We cuddled tightly—she felt so good in my arms, and it had been so long, that I tried to ignore the pain of her little body against me. Amid questions about the trapeze positioned above my bed, she rambled on about her school projects, her latest friendships, and up-and-coming birthday parties. It was a struggle not to cry as I listened, realizing how oblivious she was to what was going on, and aware that she took for granted that I would always be there for her.

I took that for granted too. We had adopted Storey when she was five months old. On the morning she arrived from Korea, I had looked down at her and felt an instant love. There was never any doubt that we would give her a good home. But I had based that faith on my continuing health and activity. Could I still offer her that good life? I hugged her tightly, and tried to quiet my doubts.

It was actually a relief to be interrupted by Jen and another couple from town, Denise and Keith, with their daughter Michelle. Though Eddie and I always felt a special closeness with Denise and Keith, it had never been more pronounced than since my accident. They inundated us with support and concern. Eddie walked back in, and just from looking at our faces, Denise and Keith knew that something was desperately wrong. I did not have to initiate the conversation, and we couldn't hide our fears from them.

The five of us talked the way you can only talk

with the best of friends; it was a much more intense conversation than any I'd been willing to have before. It was just as well, because I began to feel much better, having shared my terrible concerns with people I trusted. I *knew* they believed me.

Michelle had been clutching a bunch of daisies, which she gave to me as they left. We had talked somewhat cryptically to shelter the children. Denise and Keith suggested that, among the many options we had discussed, Eddie should contact Dr. Dupont that same day and describe the latest complications. We promised to let them know what came of the call.

Eddie dropped the girls off at his mother's and came straight back. I can remember the details of our visit that Sunday as if it were yesterday. We talked for hours. We were both frightened. We finally agreed that leaving this particular hospital environment, where no one seemed willing to take me seriously, would be a positive first step. We said good-night reluctantly, at the last call for the close of visiting hours.

Later that evening, I received a call from Jenny Adams, the owner of a nursery school in a neighboring town. I had met Jenny at the opening of her school the previous Fall. From the start, she impressed me with her creativity and enthusiasm. As we exchanged teaching philosophies, a natural chemistry developed between us. My plan had always been to return to teaching, my real career. The receptionist position was intended only as part-time work while Storey was still at home. I had made a mental note at the time to contact Jenny when Storey entered school, but Jenny beat me to it. She was calling to say that she was establishing an accredited kindergarten at her school and wanted to offer me the teaching assignment.

I was flattered and delighted by her offer, and by her confidence in me, because I recognized the high standards which she set. Kindergarten positions are rather scarce, and I find five year olds a real pleasure and challenge. The thought of being back in the classroom was really tempting. She went on to say that she felt our teaching styles were undeniably compatible. The class which she envisioned would consist of ten students, with unlimited freedom on my part for program design. It was an opportunity that would be hard to refuse.

I was in a dilemma. She obviously knew I was having some immediate medical trouble, but I'm sure she had no idea of the extent of my pain. From a selfish point of view, I wanted to say yes right then. From a professional standpoint, however, I was stuck. Teaching five year olds requires active physical participation and endless energy. Offering anything less would be unfair to the students.

I asked myself how I could even consider accepting this job offer. If I was unable to hold my four year old on my lap when I read her a story, or conduct my Brownie troop meetings for one hour a week, how could I think about teaching a class of kindergartners five days a week? My medical situation was still unsolved, and serious complications were continuing to surface.

Also, I was still officially employed at Dr. Dupont's office, and I felt a commitment to that position. I declined the offer. With mixed feelings, I wished her success in finding another candidate who would meet her needs.

When my surgeon returned the next day, my frustration surfaced uncontrollably. I accused him of taking my physical symptoms too lightly, and blurted out angrily that something had to be done. The more

I persisted that something was terribly wrong, the more emphatically the doctor insisted that no physical problem was indicated. The nurses on my floor continued to undermine my complaints. Every blood test came back normal. Examinations revealed nothing out of the ordinary. I was experiencing severe, indescribable pain, but was unable to convince my doctors. In desperation, I agreed to see the psychiatrist they recommended, hoping that another expert could influence my physicians to reconsider.

The psychiatrist initiated the discussion the next day with questions about the nature of the pain I was having. He took detailed notes to use in consulting with the other practitioners on my case. He asked whether anything unusually upsetting was occurring in my life at the time of the racquetball accident. When I told him there was nothing I could think of, he went on to ask about my relationship with my husband and children. My response was that I missed them tremendously and hated to see their visits end.

Demonstrating sincere concern, the psychiatrist explained that he was trying to determine whether this pain could be the result of a "hysterical conversion reaction," which is when a psychic conflict that has been repressed turns into a physical condition. I hoped that cooperating with him would lead to an accurate diagnosis, so I continued to answer his questions. I admit that this was difficult to do: It was humiliating to be asked if I thought the numbness and tingling in my hands could be attributed to a deeply hidden masturbation anxiety!

The psychiatrist told me that my surgeon interpreted my continual complaints as a sign that I did not want to leave the hospital. How much more wrong could these people be? What I had told the surgeon was that I did not feel comfortable leaving the hospital with more extremity pain than I had when I arrived, and without any explanation for it.

Fortunately, the psychiatrist realized that I could not wait to leave the hospital and, with his endorsement, I was discharged that same morning. I promised that I would call Dr. Dupont as soon as I got home.

I still remember the intensity of the urge to stop at the nurses' station on my way out and tell them that they were *wrong*—something really was going on in my body. I did not want to see my experience repeated with another patient. But since I had no conclusive medical findings to support my anger, I knew I would be fighting in vain. I decided to save my energy for better things.

3

Doctors and Rising Doubts

Dr. Dupont was at a loss to explain my symptoms. He suggested that I try an anti-anxiety medication and, although I was not convinced that this approach made sense, I agreed. I needed his continuing cooperation to find a valid medical explanation for my increasing pain.

As I had expected, the anxiety medication did nothing to relieve the pain. By now I was suffering with a more intense pain than I'd ever known, even during childbirth. Unlike childbirth, this affected me from head to toe.

Why couldn't I find a way to explain myself to the physicians so that they could diagnose this illness? Frustrated with my apparent inadequacy, I began to take notes on each different type of pain. I was consumed by the idea that explaining my status more clearly was the only hope I had for alleviating the discomfort which had become an everyday fact of life.

When I voluntarily scheduled a complete physical with Dr. Dupont, I realized just how sick—and frightened—I really was. As I have said, I have avoided doctors throughout much of my life. I only had physicals when they were required for school or work. This was the first time in my life that I had initiated such an appointment. The hospital from which I'd just been released did not do pre-operative exams on "healthy young women," and I was worried that some factor, some telling clue, might have been overlooked.

Dr. Dupont was fully aware of my reluctance to undergo this exam, and conducted it as quickly and considerately as he could. He listened intently as I told him that I felt like I was falling down a deep well lined with blunt steel spokes, and hitting each one, all the way down. He sensed my desperation, and drew tube after tube of blood, testing for anything that seemed even vaguely related to the symptoms I described.

Even this thorough exam resulted in a clean bill of health! The results of my CAT scan came back—normal as well. Dr. Dupont prescribed a low dosage steroid therapy. After five days on the medication, I thought I could detect a very slight improvement. But within a few more days the pain intensified, and we decided to stop the medication. Steroid treatment is risky in itself, and we agreed that we should try to avoid any unnecessary complications.

We decided to try another neurologist, to investigate the cause of the numbness and the pins-and-needles sensations. Once more, I detailed my history from the very beginning, careful not to exclude any information. The doctor shook his head sympathetically and commented on the unfortunate series of circumstances that led to having major surgery which provided no relief. His initial impression: This was definitely a matter of nerve involvement.

It is hard to express how grateful I was to have

a doctor, whose background included psychiatry, *believe me*. He had no interest in looking for a psychosomatic explanation. I went home with pain medication, counting the days until the nerve testing, scheduled for later in the week.

If ever in my life I have been sure of something, it was that this illness had a definite organic cause. Throughout my illness, out of pain and desperation, I placed an inordinate amount of hope in each test. I would listen intently to why a procedure was being ordered and what it was meant to accomplish; if it sounded at all reasonable, I found myself impatient to have it done as soon as possible. This constant expectation was frustrating—many of the tests took as long as a month to schedule, and then there was another wait for the results. When you lie awake crying all night, every night, with penetrating pain throughout your body, a month can seem like a year. I feel sorry that some of you reading this story can identify with this physical and emotional state. It is a terrible form of suffering.

The day of my test finally arrived—snowy and threatening. I was anxious about driving in the bad weather, but more anxious to have the test done. I detailed my increased pain and limited mobility to the doctor, who seemed to share my sense of urgency about solving this puzzle.

The nerve test was unlike any I'd had before. The neurologist applied a stimulus at a point on my skin, and my reaction was immediately recorded and compared against a table of normal reaction times. All the readings measured within normal limits.

The neurologist chose to pursue another lead. He knew that I had been hospitalized three years prior to my injury for a large white cell (CMV) virus which had stayed with me for months. He speculated that the virus might never have left my system. He also thought it was possible that the trauma of the racquetball accident might have triggered the virus from a latent to an active state. This virus might be attacking the nerves around my spinal column.

I was placed on erythromycin, the antibiotic which had been effective earlier in treating the virus. Considering the other, more traumatic diagnoses that had been suggested, a virus was something I'd almost welcome. I prayed that the pills would work. I took them for two weeks, with no positive results.

My next step was to go back to Dr. Dupont, and the details of this visit remain with me even amid the swirl of doctors and tests. He patiently reviewed the results of all the bloodwork he had done and explained the negative results of each test. Nothing was adding up. He offered to send me to a teaching hospital for further evaluation on the condition that I talk to another psychiatrist, to determine once and for all whether the problem was psychosomatic.

I argued with him: I had just seen a neurologist with a specialty in psychiatry who agreed that there was an organic root to this pain. My doctor remained adamant. I was so upset that I didn't know what to do next. I agreed to see the psychiatrist he had in mind only because I knew I would need his support to get into the teaching hospital. As I walked out the door, he told me to have a good month. Though I didn't say it, I knew I wouldn't have a good day, month, or year until an accurate diagnosis was made and appropriate treatment started.

Confused, angry, and feeling letdown, I drove to my friend Diane's house. We had known each other since college, and although we didn't see each other very often, the same closeness was always there. When I saw her car in the driveway, I started to cry, desperate to talk with a real friend. She made me a cup of coffee as I told her about the no-win ultimatum I felt I had been given: See another psychiatrist or forfeit the chance to be evaluated at the teaching hospital.

What choice did I have? My pain was unbearable. I couldn't find a comfortable position in any chair at Diane's house, and felt myself grimace each time I shifted my weight. While Diane agreed that it was an unfair situation, she also believed that seeing the psychiatrist would be my quickest route to a higher level of evaluation, with a variety of specialists. I felt much better emotionally, if not physically, by the time I headed home.

My initial visit with the psychiatrist went about as I had expected. She was easy to talk to and asked sensible questions, which were not as upsetting or as extreme as in the earlier evaluation. The only negative memory I have is of the constant discomfort I felt sitting for an hour at a time. I saw her twice, and at the end of our second session she informed me that my doctor should continue to look for a physical source for my problems.

Dr. Dupont received her report with confidence, but by now many other specialists were associated with my case. Another of these physicians was of the opinion that the psychiatrist "might have missed something," and asked that I go back a third time. Basically, I used this session to explain why I felt this doctor's hunch was wrong.

I discussed with Dr. Dupont every disease that even vaguely resembled my situation. I feared multiple sclerosis and questioned him extensively about it, though he had been confident from the onset of the illness that I did not have MS because my symptoms differed from those of MS patients he was already treating. He set up, as he had promised, an appointment at the nearby teaching hospital, where I was to be evaluated by a neuromuscular specialist. The examination would probably include a spinal tap, which was often used to identify MS.

My work status, as you might imagine, had changed significantly by this time. I had not worked since shortly after the accident. Though I repeatedly asked to return, hoping that work could provide a distraction from the now constant pain, some of my employers were concerned that the strong pain medication I was taking could affect my judgment. They worried about me making mistakes on the job. Given that I was unable to function without the pain medication, there was no room for compromise.

In the midst of all the testing, I heard from Jenny Adams, who again offered me the teaching position. Stubbornly—and undoubtedly foolishly—I decided to consider it. I was in no condition to work, but I refused to admit it.

I went to the school to observe for a day, and found that I could hardly walk. My arms and legs burned as though they were on fire. I forced myself to ignore the pain, and concentrated on the bubbling, enthusiastic children. I tried to join the children who were practicing a marching routine for a parents' program, and finally just had to sit down. I *couldn't* ignore the pain. Working to hold back my tears, I left for home.

The school's director phoned that evening, eager for my first impressions. While I was enthusiastic about the school, I had to admit to her that I was not doing well physically. She invited me to an open house the following month, where, if I felt up to it, I could speak to the parents and meet prospective students. I agreed to that, ever hopeful, but asked her not to introduce me as the kindergarten teacher. It would be unfair to lead the children to believe that I might be their teacher, when there was a good chance that I would not be able to accept the position.

The open house turned out to be a sizable event. Maybe the director was overly enthusiastic, or perhaps she had forgotten our agreement, but she introduced me as the teacher she was hoping would say yes to the kindergarten position. This led to a deluge of questions from the parents regarding my goals, background, and philosophy. I was enjoying every minute! It felt tremendous to be back in an educational environment. . . but the constant discomfort I felt was an ominous reminder of the reality of my situation.

With my symptoms worsening even as I left the gathering, I was troubled that Jenny was depending on me to accept the position. I had procrastinated long enough and called her that night to decline. I explained that, from a professional standpoint, it was the only choice I could make. Although my heart wasn't in it, I had to say no because of my health. She understood that my decision was final, and did not try to change my mind. We promised to keep in touch. I was confident as I hung up the phone that I had made the only logical decision—but that did not make my disappointment any easier to live with.

Eddie came with me a few days later to the post-surgical visit with the neurosurgeon who had operated on my back. Because my symptoms had continued to intensify despite the surgery, we were understandably concerned. The surgeon was obviously perplexed as he repeated the neurological exam. He recommended that I see the neurologist who had been called in to consult during my hospitalization. I was completely unenthusiastic about the idea, remembering how uncomfortable I had been with him. I was tired of agreeing to tests out of desperation.

When I returned to the consulting neurologist, he repeated many of the questions and tests that we had gone through in the hospital. I could have done the tests in my sleep by now. When his findings again came out negative, he concluded that the more sophisticated tests recommended by the referring doctor were not indicated, and instead wrote out a prescription "to help me sleep."

I called Dr. Dupont as soon as I got home and told him the name of the medication prescribed. He told me that the neurologist probably suspected my problem was a simple case of nerves. With Dr. Dupont's endorsement, I refused to take the medicine, and decided that I would never see that neurologist again.

I stopped by Diane's, ready for some decent conversation; by now she was used to my impromptu visits. Much to my surprise, she seemed for the first time to doubt that I was going to find a medical explanation. I listened in disbelief, with my stomach beginning to ache, as she demanded that I "look at the facts": all my tests were negative. I started to understand, watching her face and hearing her change the topic whenever I talked about the illness, that she had come to agree with the doctors.

I was overwhelmed; I had to get out of her house. I left as fast as my sore leg muscles would allow and burst into tears standing in the driveway. This was no longer that slow trickle of reluctant tears I used to let through, but hard, shaking sobbing. Diane was one of the people I could count on when the odds were stacked against me. I needed her now more than ever, as my body grew weaker. But she stopped the daily calls, which she, like Jen, had made since my first hospital visit. On the increasingly rare occasions when we saw each other, she pointedly chose *not* to ask how I was doing.

Diane was the most important, but not the only friend who doubted me. Many of my friends showed skepticism about the validity of my symptoms. Some became less available. Several pointed out that the clinical findings did not support my continued "complaints." A few said they had talked to other friends who assured them that I was "just fine," and that there was nothing wrong with me. Others offered impractical suggestions like taking hot showers, though I had explained that I could not even stand up in the shower. Some criticized me for not considering my family's needs, when I questioned whether I could sit through the four-hour drive to the Cape for our annual vacation.

I can't imagine not being there for them if the situation were reversed. But then, I knew just how severe the pain was because I lived with it; they didn't. Fortunately, throughout this long period I had the continued support of a small group of friends who consistently believed that a physical explanation would be found. They stood by me and my family, against popular opinion, and to this day are central to my ability to cope with my changing life.

4

False Leads

When Dr. Dupont requested an appointment with the teaching hospital, we were told that I could not be given one before May, which was nearly a month away. I made another call myself, explaining my urgent need for an evaluation, the months of inconclusive tests, and all the ways in which I would be forced to cut back, including forfeiting our vacation on the Cape if I still did not know what was wrong. The appointment was moved up by two weeks. Though pleased with my success in changing the appointment, advocating for myself was becoming more and more exhausting.

Dr. Dupont was away for a few days when I noticed that my vision was becoming blurred. I called an associate in the office to report this, and he called back later after looking over the results of several blood tests done earlier in the week. There was obviously something wrong; his voice was *very* serious. The tests had shown an abnormal anti-nuclear antibody (ANA) level, which could be indicative of a connective tissue disease, such as lupus.

These are serious illnesses. Lupus, he explained,

is an autoimmune disorder which can affect every part of the body. He decided to put me back on steroids, at a higher dosage than I'd taken before. He also prescribed a sleep-inducing medication that had been successful with connective tissue diseases. Finally, he ordered more bloodwork, to eliminate the chance of a lab error.

My mind was racing. Could this mean that we were finally on to something, after all these months? If so, what was wrong, and how bad would it be? I vacillated between fear that I had something terribly serious and relief that I was on the verge of a diagnosis and possibly a cure.

After a week on the steroid medication, I noticed a decrease in my pain. Then, as I stepped out of bed one morning, my legs collapsed under me. Eddie, on the other side of the room, only had time to turn and look on helplessly as I fell down hard to the floor.

I had feared paralysis since the start of the illness, and had often asked Dr. Dupont if he suspected that the leg pain and numbness might lead to this. The fall brought all my worst fears to the surface. But the doctor attributed the fall to the sleep-inducing medication and immediately discontinued it.

A few days later, I got a call telling me that the latest bloodwork showed a *normal* ANA level; the earlier result must have been an error. I wish it had occurred to me at the time to ask how we could be sure that the *second* test was the accurate one. The doctor immediately decided to discontinue the steroid treatment.

I argued with him; my pain had decreased on this medication. For the first time since the accident, I had seen some real improvement in the quality of my daily life. He countered that it would be dangerous to remain on a powerful drug without a conclusive blood test. How do lab errors like this occur? How many other patients experience these medical inconsistencies, at the expense of their health and peace of mind?

Eddie, Storey, and I headed for the teaching hospital some days later, grateful that the date had finally arrived. We speculated hopefully about the appointment, whiling away the time in the car and attempting to reinforce our confidence that we were doing the right thing.

The neuromuscular specialist was empathetic and straightforward. I related the whole story again, which I was beginning to feel I should have taped, so I could just push a button whenever we needed to replay what was by now months of information.

The doctor conducted another standard neurological exam, emphasizing pinpricks and buzzing sensations, and checking my directional awareness with my eyes closed. Once again, my responses were normal.

I didn't argue when the doctor called in a rheumatologist to consult on my case. This man noted that my fingers and toes were slightly blue, and asked if this was a common occurrence. I had to admit that I had never noticed it, and even then did not find the color obvious. The two doctors, however, felt it was significant, and again ordered what seemed to be every blood test imaginable. I warned them that the results would be negative and, after a full morning of exams, promised to return the next week for muscle tests.

Any remaining positive effects from the steroids had by now worn off, and again I spent most nights awake, in severe pain. Because I lacked sleep so desperately, it was next to impossible to handle anything approaching a normal day's activities. My doctors were opposed to any strong pain medication.

Those who felt that this was not an organic problem feared I would become addicted. I had to rely on Eddie and my friends to do grocery shopping, cooking, and driving. I finally had to admit to myself that I could not even hold a wrap-up meeting for my Brownie troop. These may sound like small concessions, but they amounted to giving up a substantial part of my world—I could not give or receive in many of the ways that had meant the most to me.

When I went back for the muscle testing, the neurologist commented on how serious I looked. Of course I looked serious! None of this was fun. I did not understand what was happening to me and I was not getting any answers. I had run out of adjectives to describe my increasing pain. I had only one priority, and it was a serious one!

This testing was actually interesting, though more uncomfortable than some of the other studies. The doctor inserted needles into various muscles and observed my muscle strength and activity on a monitor. He also ran more nerve conduction studies.

When the results all came out normal, the rheumatologist and neurologist agreed that my pain was due to a condition called fibrositis, or muscular rheumatism. Although this condition could create severe muscle pain throughout the body, it was not as serious a disease as some of the others we had discussed. Exercise, they informed me, is the best remedy. I tried to convey, again, how difficult everyday motions had become, let alone any kind of serious exercise. There were times when I was unable to hold my thirty-five pound daughter on my lap. Handshakes were excruciating and walking was worse. It was painful just to be touched.

While the neurologist empathized, he explained that my problem was more rheumatological than neurological. That is, the illness most likely involved muscles and connective tissue, rather than nerves. His advice was to select a rheumatologist close to my home and see him or her on a regular basis. The other advice he gave me was to avoid steroids, if at all possible, because of their many harmful side effects. He recommended trying other drugs first. Given his sincere interest in me, in contrast to some of the other attitudes I'd encountered, I left wishing that he could remain on my case.

Shortly after my visit, I had an occasion to bring Storey to her physician for a minor problem. In response to his inquiry about my condition, I explained the fibrositis diagnosis to him. He commented on how relieved I must be to have a name for my condition; wouldn't this make it all easier to live with?

While he exclaimed that I was lucky it was "nothing serious," I kept my silence, wondering how willing he would be to accept this diagnosis if he could appreciate the intensity of my pain. I was hesitant to settle for this latest "answer." I knew there was much more to come.

I contacted Dr. Dupont for a referral to a local rheumatologist. I said I wanted a competent, caring specialist, someone I could work with effectively on a long-term basis. I was tired of "doctor-hopping."

Without hesitation, he recommended a specialist nearby, and I understood his certainty about Dr. Michaels as soon as we met. He immediately made me feel comfortable and listened intently as I described my history, asking questions, but allowing enough time for me to give a good description of each event. When I'd finished, he looked at me very seriously and told me that I was *not* describing fibrositis. Instead, he felt I had something far more involved, active throughout my body—probably a connective tissue disease. A chill of fear went through me when he asked whether any of my physicians had mentioned the possibility of multiple sclerosis or lupus. They had, of course, and I'd lived with these fears, but again and again I had been told that I did not have one of these more serious diseases.

I was shaking as we went into the examining room. I suppose I should have been relieved to see that someone was getting close to the source of my pain, but on the other hand, this was a far cry from what had appeared five months ago to be a pulled muscle. Suddenly I found myself wishing it *were* a psychological problem, which we could solve through counseling. I was getting closer to what I'd said I wanted—a diagnosis—but I was also terribly afraid.

He performed a thorough physical, including an EKG and joint and muscle strength tests. Back in his office, he wrote out a prescription for pain medication; I needed all my strength to fight this illness, and he recognized that I wasn't doing well without sleep. He also pointed out that some diseases took a very long time to register any clinical results. We decided that I would be monitored every three weeks, with the understanding that I would let him know immediately if any significant changes occurred. If any rashes or swelling appeared, I was to come in at once. My visits with him would supplement those with Dr. Dupont.

I cannot describe the reassurance I felt because of this doctor's confidence in me. After some of the horrendous experiences I had had with physicians who did not believe that I was sick, I welcomed his conviction that the illness had an organic basis. He gave me some pamphlets on tic bites and various types of arthritis, asking that I review them in terms of my illness. My symptoms were so clear to me that it was an easy process to eliminate these possibilities, but the point is that he trusted me to do this, without expecting that I might imagine myself a candidate for every disease I read about. Following his advice, I continued to see him every three weeks, took the pain medication, and lived a very scaled-down life.

Dr. Michaels referred me at one point to a dermatologist for a skin biopsy, to see if this would reveal conclusive evidence of a connective tissue disorder. The procedure itself was simple—the removal of a small section of skin from the back of my hand for lab analysis. This was performed in the doctor's office, and only a few stitches were required. It was no more traumatic than having a cavity filled.

The dermatologist was interested in my case. He examined my hands, which at the time were turning blue. He recorded a diagnosis of Raynaud's phenomenon—a circulatory problem I had first heard mentioned by the rheumatologist at the teaching hospital.

A note of further frustration comes to mind on this count. Though three doctors had by that time recorded Raynaud's phenomenon as one of my symptoms, when I reported this to another physician, he claimed that this was not a part of my illness. Short of following physicians around 24 hours a day, revealing each new phenomenon as it happened, how could I convince them of the *facts* of my case? Why weren't the written opinions of three doctors enough? This kind of disregard for cumulative evidence was a definite deterrent to obtaining a final diagnosis.

At the end of a week of waiting for my biopsy results, I received a call telling me—guess what? Completely normal. Although discouraged not to be any closer to an answer, I was again relieved that no serious disease had been uncovered.

Dr. Michaels was confused as to why the pain remained so persistent. As a next step, he suggested a sural nerve biopsy. By removing a one-inch section of this nerve from the bottom of my foot, the surgeon could scrutinize tissue that appeared to be consistently involved. Vein and muscle sections could also be analyzed. Some of the diseases which I feared most, including multiple sclerosis, could be detected from this type of biopsy. It all seemed logical, if frightening, and I contacted a surgeon to discuss the procedure.

5

Sural Nerve Biopsy

I went to my appointment on a steamy, too-thick-to-breathe July afternoon. The surgeon's waiting room was cool to the point of being frigid, and it had a standing room only crowd. I had to assume these people had been waiting a long time; they rolled their eyes and tapped their feet, looking exasperated or bored. I settled against a wall lined with brochures and listened to the typical office music being piped in. My legs were not holding up well, and just at the moment that I was sure I was going to collapse, several names were called and I slid into a chair.

The surgeon was a tall, thin woman, with a thick accent that I found difficult to negotiate. She took a medical history more brief than I was used to and went straight into the physical exam. She seemed to be particularly interested in any evidence of circulatory problems. Finding nothing along that line, she theorized that my symptoms were probably due to vein spasticity caused by coffee consumption! At the time, I was only drinking one or two cups of decaffeinated coffee a day. Once again, I had been sent to a physician who did not understand the serious nature of my symptoms and, in this case, was simply not listening.

What an underreaction to the facts of my case. It only caused my fear and frustration to work overtime to have these experts misunderstand what I tried so hard to convey. It was more stressful for me to consider the many diseases that I *might* have than it would have been to let the medical profession narrow it down for me, no matter how bad the diagnosis proved to be.

The surgeon matter-of-factly informed me that the two things I did *not* want this to be were MS or a connective tissue disease. I was at a loss to respond to such a depressing and negative statement, knowing that either diagnosis was quite possible. She insisted that we were not dealing with anything "that serious," but the thought kept going through my mind, what if she is wrong, and I have one of the diseases that she considers next to hopeless? I tried to console myself, remembering that other physicians had said that these more serious diseases were only disabling in a minority of severe cases. As I sat there, I told myself: You will be able to function, whatever the outcome.

The surgeon described the nerve biopsy for me, which would involve a one-inch incision on my left foot. She would also do a muscle biopsy at the same time. Her only surgical concern was that the procedure might result in permanent numbness in a small portion of my foot. I was unconcerned; my other doctors had told me that the area involved was so minuscule it would not affect my walking or general activity. While I was uncertain about *this* surgeon, I was confident that my doctors felt the procedure was worthwhile, and the best choice I had for the moment. I also hoped that the biopsy would tell us whether I had vasculitis—a possibility mentioned by several doctors, involving the inflammation and degeneration of blood vessels.

The surgeon's parting comment was a shock: She bluntly let me know that she was *opposed* to doing the biopsy and expected nothing diagnostically significant to come from it. Her negativity intimidated me so much that I was at a complete loss for words.

I went out into the humid summer air and sat in my car. The longer I sat there, the more unsettled I became about going through with the biopsy. My body had been poked and dissected more than enough; I certainly did not need unnecessary surgery. When I got home, I called another physician, who reminded me of all the good reasons for the procedure. His encouragement helped me decide to have it done.

My friend Sue offered to take care of the girls, and at first I refused. Considering the minor nature of the biopsy, her help did not seem necessary. I had had no difficulty recovering from surgeries in the past; this one should be a snap. Her deep concern for us as a family and her understanding of the stress we were under finally convinced me. Her help was simply a generous guarantee that I would not be overly troubled by this latest disruption.

I registered that next Monday as an outpatient at a hospital about an hour away. The preliminary surgical procedures were uneventful. When the anesthesiologist asked me how I felt, I confided that I was apprehensive about the exploratory nature of the surgery, and anxious because of the serious diseases that might be diagnosed. He remarked, as the surgeon entered the room, that though I was well-prepared for the surgery, I certainly had legitimate concerns. The surgeon suddenly became very animated and asserted that I *should* be concerned, given that I might be left with permanent damage to my foot, and could have trouble walking. That was the first I'd heard of that possibility! I started to shake uncontrollably.

The surgeon asked me whose word I was going to take, hers or that of an internist? She let me know again that she was not in favor of removing part of the sural nerve, and hastily scrawled out a statement witnessing that the surgical risks had been explained to me. I signed the paper, although I could hardly see to write through the tears filling my eyes. What was I getting myself into? Would I be able to walk normally? Why did she wait until now to tell me this? Were the other doctors keeping things from me?

I was terrified by the implications of all that had been said, and felt all alone in the cold room. I wanted Eddie there. I wanted to talk to Dr. Michaels. Instead, I was on my way into exploratory surgery . . . with an uncertain outcome.

As the surgeon left the room, she asked which foot was to be operated on. I responded automatically: the left. And a moment later felt the question shatter what little was left of my confidence. The doctor had to ask *me* which foot to work on?

Having overheard the surgeon's remarks, the anesthesiologist went out of his way to reassure me as we walked to the operating room. But I was too upset to appreciate his efforts. I tried to hold down that salty feeling in my throat that meant I was about to be sick, and laid down on the cold metal table, under the bright round lights. There were shining steel instruments all around me. I told the anesthesiologist that I just wanted to be put under, and have the whole thing over with.

The next thing I recognized was the sound of loud voices calling my name, through what seemed a hollow, echoing tunnel. Masked faces came into view and the anesthesiologist informed me that the surgery had not yet started because the doctor needed to verify which foot to operate on. Even in my half-sleep, this seemed absurd. For the second time that day, I reminded her that it was the left foot. I was put back to sleep, exasperated and afraid.

My next recollection was opening my eyes as the anesthesiologist wheeled me out of the operating room. My leg throbbed; I had a large gauze wrap around my foot, ankle, and part of my leg. The surgeon came in to say that it had taken two incisions to ensure the least loss of nerve sensation. No wonder my leg hurt. That also explained the huge bandage.

Her preliminary report: Though the biopsies were not back yet, nothing abnormal was observed during the procedure. I felt no more reassured than before the surgery. The question of MS was still unanswered. Connective tissue disease had not been ruled out. We were dealing with serious illnesses, and my diagnosis was still up in the air. I was afraid to consider what the final outcome would be, but at the same time I was desperate to know. This entire illness had been one progressive nightmare.

After the required two-hour stay, when I'd been fortified with toast and coffee, it was time to leave. Or was it? When I tried to stand, I felt a penetrating pain in my ankle. The incision began to ooze and wouldn't stop. It was next to impossible to put any weight on my foot.

The nurses immediately offered me crutches, but I responded stubbornly. I was not about to look anything like an invalid. I didn't want any more attention drawn to me. And I just could not justify leaving the hospital on crutches, when I had been told this was a simple outpatient procedure.

When Eddie arrived, he also tried to convince me that the crutches would help. In retrospect, I can see that fear was the controlling factor in my irrational behavior. I had an intuition that this was a debilitating disease, and using crutches made that possibility into a reality. My refusal was an ineffective attempt to put up a fight, to have some *control*—even if it was only saying no to those crutches. I had always prided myself on being an independent person, and I planned to remain one until I no longer had a choice.

Armed with pain medication and a lot of willful pride, I left the hospital. I remember trying to resist when Eddie offered his arm. I wanted to make it from that conspicuous wheelchair to the car by myself, but I had to give in.

When I got home, I propped up my throbbing foot and leg. I was surprised by the intensity of the pain from these small incisions, and grateful to Sue for insisting on taking the girls. This discomfort was much greater than what I had felt after the disk surgery a few months earlier.

When the hospital's outpatient department called the next day to check on me, I let them know how much pain I was in, and that I was shocked that this surgery was performed as an outpatient procedure. The nurse seemed perplexed, and suggested that I report the situation to my doctor. My stitches were to be removed on Friday; I decided I could hold out until then. I told Eddie that I was going to be very embarrassed if, when the bandages were removed, I only had a few tiny stitches. I limped through the week, spending most of each day in bed.

On Friday, I explained to the surgeon's nurse that I was still in considerable pain, and that putting any weight on my leg caused the incision to leak. She raised an eyebrow and looked quite skeptical, but

when she unwrapped the bandage her look of amazement could not be disguised. Through squinting eyes,
like a little child trying to avoid seeing something, I
looked down and saw more scarring on my leg than I
had had from my back surgery. There was a three-
inch incision on my ankle and a smaller one on my
leg, all held together with at least 20 staples.

I wish I had answered assertively when the surgeon came in and asked me what I thought. I wish I'd
had the nerve to tell her what I really felt. This was a
far cry from a one-inch incision on the bottom of my
foot.

Instead, intimidated by whatever bad news she
might give me, I told her only that I was not pleased
and that I had not expected anything like this. I
offered my amazement that this was done as an outpatient procedure.

She explained that I probably should have been
admitted, given that the surgery was more involved
than she had anticipated. She had made the decision
to send me home because she felt I could handle the
recovery stage successfully.

I resented her unilateral, secretive decision. I had
spent the last five days basically immobile, getting up
only to go to the bathroom, and then having to shuf-
fle or hop on my right leg, which had pains of its
own. The least she could have done was fill me in,
prepare me. My face was hot with anger. (Later, I
wondered whether my flush was more than anger;
was it a clue to my diagnosis?) The incisions had not
healed enough for the stitches to be removed; I would
have to return the next week.

Although my mobility increased during the week,
the incisions continued to leak and throb. And my
overall, undiagnosed pain was becoming worse. Our
Cape Cod vacation was scheduled, but packing for it

seemed monumental. I began to doubt whether I would be able to go, but tried again and again to convince myself that I would feel better once I got there and could relax.

By Friday I was feeling like a perpetual patient. I was followed into the examining room by the doctor, her nurse, and a resident. As the resident began removing the staples, the surgeon stopped her. The incisions had not healed. I was infuriated. After almost two weeks, this "minor outpatient procedure" was still not finished. The staples that had been taken out prematurely left raw areas that I would have to apply steri strips to daily.

The biopsy and other test results had all come back negative. I had reason to be elated, I suppose, but as I looked down at my disfigured leg, I could only think that this surgery had been for nothing. I knew I was not out of the woods. None of our questions had been answered, and I still did not know what I had or how to treat my increasing pain.

The surgeon tried to convince me that I should be relieved that the very serious diseases which might have been found had been "disproved." She was pleased with the outcome.

On my way home, I dropped in on Sue. I was so angry I couldn't see straight. I recited to her the twenty-minute reproach I'd been too intimidated to give the surgeon. It felt so good to be able to release some of that accumulating anger. I was grateful to have such an empathetic listener.

6

Family Matters

I was ready to get away. I *needed* this vacation, and so did Eddie and the girls. It was late July, and it had been so long since we'd been able to relax together.

Everyone knew from the outset that some of our usual activities were in jeopardy. Eddie and I had told the girls that I would not be able to come with them on our traditional bike rides and walks along the beach. We were only slightly discouraged, though: Cape Cod is a very special place to each of us, full of carefree memories.

Eddie bought me a comfortable sand chair, and we visited a bookstore where I stocked up on two weeks' worth of good reading. I was looking forward to a stretch of time for reading. Stacey and Storey were touching in their efforts to find substitute projects for me, as they planned for all their regular vacation sports.

Although Storey frequently asked how I was feeling, she was young enough to remain oblivious to many of our worries. However, my illness was taking its toll emotionally on our eight year old, Stacey. She began having recurring nightmares and was walking in her sleep. In her dreams, I had died and her father had to take both daughters to work with him each morning. It was a reasonable guess at the future, from a child's point of view. We had been careful to keep her informed about my illness and had always answered her questions honestly, but now Eddie and I realized she needed some professional reassurance.

Just before we left for the Cape, we took Stacey to her physician. The two of them had a warm and friendly relationship, and the visit proved invaluable. She told him her fears that I might die, or have cancer and have to live in a hospital for the rest of my life. She expressed her doubt that there could be a happy outcome, when the doctors could not say what was wrong. As I watched her eyes fill with tears, I was reminded of what a nightmare these months had been for *all* of us, and I cried too. While no one else felt the physical pain, each of us shared in the emotional struggle.

The doctor was terrific, encouraging Stacey to talk about the ways in which her life had changed since I became ill. (In truth, through a lot of determination and cooperation from Eddie and our friends, the girls' activities had changed only minimally.) He explained that while no one knew yet what illness I had, the test results did not show that I was going to die. There was only a small chance that my illness was cancer-related, and he told her that while I might have to go into a hospital for short periods, I would not have to live there.

The doctor complimented us on keeping Stacey so well informed and described her feelings as a very natural extension of my fears. This made a lot of sense to me. I was scared and it was reasonable that she would pick up on my feelings. He made sure that Stacey knew she could call him if she thought of any other questions. We left with a much-relieved child, who has not had a nightmare or a sleepwalking incident since.

We spent our first week at Cape Cod in absolutely beautiful weather. But a perfect setting and plenty of relaxation did not make my symptoms disappear. One evening we had to leave a scrumptious dinner when my legs began to hurt so much that I couldn't remain composed. I became weak trying to get in and out of the low lawn chairs, and could walk for only a minute or two before being forced by the pain to sit down again. The incision on my leg was still partly open, which meant frequent cleaning and sterilizing. Even with around-the-clock medication, the pain intensified.

My brother and my husband's sister and family arrived at the end of the first week. My brother had a scared, sad look in his eyes throughout his stay, particularly when I was at my worst. He continually offered help with cooking, and assisted me in getting around. My sister-in-law quickly saw that I was in more pain than ever, and she was a tremendous help, too. Yet even though I was *literally* doing nothing, I felt worse every day. I took as much pain medication as was allowed, far more than I'd been taking, and still could not sleep.

Some of my reluctance to make this trip had been based on the fear of being isolated from the doctors familiar with my case. What would I do if my condition worsened? Now these worries were becoming reality. I didn't want to find a doctor on Cape Cod and explain the whole story again. On the other hand, maybe there was some significance to my condition changing so dramatically this week. Could the sun or the dampness have had a negative effect? Was I only imagining that I was beginning to lose hair, or was this a new symptom of the disease? Midway through the second week, I was becoming desperate.

One afternoon, after about half an hour in the sun, I broke out in a rash on my upper back. It was red and didn't itch, so it was not sun poisoning. It lasted all day. I wished that it would have appeared when I was home and the doctors had asked about rashes. They had asked frequently, so I knew that this had some diagnostic significance. I tried to watch it closely, so I could describe it confidently at my next appointment.

While thinking about all this, I suddenly remembered attending a woman's club meeting several years earlier, where two lupus patients spoke about their disease. They distributed pamphlets and books about lupus, and I recalled being very inattentive, feeling that "that only happens to other people." Then I remembered them speaking about a sun-sensitive rash, and knew that I needed to go to the library as soon as I got home, to educate myself about lupus. The doctors had found no clear evidence that this was lupus, but I was very suspicious.

The vacation had ceased to be at all enjoyable. We decided to leave early—a decision I was later glad I made. I was anxious to describe the latest symptoms to Dr. Dupont, and hopeful that they might lead to an accurate diagnosis. Also, I had an appointment at another teaching hospital, which had an excellent reputation with connective tissue diseases. Once again, I became hopeful that I was about to learn why I was so ill.

7

Another Teaching Hospital

When I got home from the Cape, I found a lengthy preliminary questionnaire from the teaching hospital. I spent several hours filling it out, and mailed away the bulky envelope, my fingers cramped and throbbing. When I arrived at the hospital two weeks later, I was asked several times to describe my medical history. I had to question whether composing all those essays—a literally painful exercise—had been completely in vain.

A third-year resident assigned to my case was the first to volunteer that I displayed many of the characteristics of a lupus patient. He was particularly interested in the rash I'd developed at the Cape. He based his conjecture on the sun sensitivity in combination with the overall muscle pain and general weakness.

Insisting that he was only speculating, the resident assured me that the rheumatologist I was scheduled to see had extensive experience with lupus and so was very well qualified to analyze my symptoms. The resident went on to conduct a standard physical exam, as I lamented to myself that I had done more than my share for the future physicians of America.

Dr. Burke, the rheumatologist, demonstrated real concern and empathy right from the start. I repeated my story as she conducted a supplemental exam. Looking perplexed, she said that she understood why the other physicians were confused by the case: Although many of my symptoms corresponded with a connective tissue disease, such as lupus, others did not. Even the symptoms which pointed to lupus were not appearing in a typical manner. Lupus, for example, can cause sun sensitivity, but this usually appears as a "butterfly" pattern across the patient's face.

As if reading my mind, Dr. Burke acknowledged how difficult it must be to present a clear, detailed history and still not have a diagnosis, or even an appropriate treatment program. Because of the idiosyncrasies of my case, she wanted to present it at the departmental meeting scheduled for that afternoon; a brainstorming session among several physicians might uncover a connection.

I had, again, put high hopes into this visit, and she must have sensed my disappointment when she told me I would have to wait three days for any results. Gently, she pointed out that I had been ill for eight months now and had managed to confuse a dozen doctors; surely I couldn't expect her to have all the answers on her first evaluation. Rationally, I saw her point. But, selfishly, I didn't have to like it. The wait for her phone call seemed like an eternity. Everyone asked about the results of the visit, but I had no answers, only continuing head to toe pain. The pain medication was becoming less effective.

When she called, she had nothing earth-shattering to report from the joint meeting, but the doctors did have a few ideas. They wanted to admit me to rule out the possibility of MS, brain infection, or trichinosis, which can be mistaken for rheumatism. I called Dr. Dupont to give him the news, and confided that I felt like a guinea pig. I was afraid of this next round.

At 11:00 on Monday morning, Eddie delivered me, hopeful and apprehensive, to the admitting area. With a quick kiss and a promise to stop by that evening, he left for work. My suitcase was bulging with my standard essentials and plenty of books. Within half an hour I was in a cheerful, semi-private room, trying to make myself at home.

As I hung up my robe, a nurse came in to begin what would be a nonstop series of interviews, going on until 5:00 that evening. Nurses, dieticians, interns, and doctors made rounds. Repeatedly, I detailed the history of my illness, beginning with the racquetball accident and ending with a description of the pulsating muscular pain I now felt continuously. I tried to recall anything that might be significant and outlined the results of each test and doctor's opinion. Something just had to click.

In addition to the interviews, there were numerous exams. I began to cringe at the sound of the curtain being pulled along the metal rod encircling my bed. Medical students seem to conduct the longest, most involved exams. They invariably say that they are there to conduct a "brief" exam, but it never is. When I began to worry to myself about how many more of these exams I might have to endure, my thoughts switched over to how terribly painful the past eight months had been. That image alone was enough to convince me that I could undergo a hundred more physicals with a hundred more doctors if it would alleviate even a portion of my pain. I had to come to the end of this mystery.

Eddie was a welcome sight at the end of a fatiguing day. I unloaded all my feelings onto him—no matter how many details I remembered, no one knew what was wrong. I had driven myself, night after night, through tears that soaked my pillow, to find more exact ways to describe the pain I felt. If these descriptions still weren't enough to reach a diagnosis, it certainly wasn't my fault.

Eddie and I talked through dinner. He was concerned, of course, but also optimistic that I was at last in the right place. This hopeful attitude had carried us through each new medical endeavor, and it surfaced again as we spoke. Just then, Dr. Burke stopped by to describe the tests she had ordered and what she hoped to learn. Eddie found her confidence reassuring, and we agreed that her approach made sense.

Eddie left to pick up Storey from a friend's home. Stacey was at camp all week and unaware that I was in the hospital. Remembering her earlier apprehension, we thought that sparing her any more unpleasant news would be best.

I lost myself in a good book, until I was distracted by voices outside my door at about 10:00 p.m. Whatever it was, couldn't it wait until morning? I heard a medical student talking to a resident, asking if he needed gloves for the procedure he was about to perform. A lump formed in my throat as I realized that this unsure student was about to do his first spinal tap, on me! The thought of this young man's inexperience made me shiver.

My fears were not unrealistic. The procedure dragged on and the student's many attempts were unsuccessful, even with additional injections of novocaine. Finally the resident took over and completed the procedure, promising to let the student try again on someone who had no scar tissue. They teased me as they left the room: Sure you're going to make it? My fear of becoming a guinea pig had been well founded.

Early the next morning a neurologist came in for a consultation. He explained that he had been summoned on the chance that some degeneration of my nervous system was involved. He wanted to let me know that, based on the examinations and tests performed, I certainly did not have either a brain tumor or a hemorrhage. Those were fears I could put to rest. His visit was quite a relief.

The hospital room was becoming all too familiar, and I was bored. I decided to take a walk in the hall. Within two minutes I had to turn around, unable to put weight on my legs any longer. I was greeted in my room by several residents and a medical student. They had come to share their dilemma with me. They admitted that even with all the testing that had been done, they did not have a clue as to what was wrong with me. As expected, my bloodwork was normal. All my organs were functioning properly.

Seeing my obvious discomfort as I lowered myself into a seat, they asked where I was hurting, which happened to be in my right thigh. I was also experiencing a strong burning sensation in my left arm. They left the room shaking their heads and conferring. I tried to settle down into my book, but I was distracted by that terribly disappointing pronouncement.

I was still staring at the pages of my book when I overheard a conversation that was much more disturbing. For nearly an hour, the voices of these same residents, the medical student, and the senior physician echoed from a nearby hallway into my room. They were reviewing *my* case. The residents spoke about their frustration at being unable to reach a diagnosis. They emphasized the severity of my pain and its chronic nature, and pointed out that I had been perfectly healthy before the accident. They reminded the physician of the details which I had recounted to them all: transient, blurry vision, severe extremity pain, hair loss, abnormally strong reflex responses, and "pins and needles" numbness on the soles of my feet as well as my hands, lips, tongue, and the roof of my mouth. They described, as I had to them, the pulsating sensation that I experienced throughout my body.

The senior physician's reaction was infuriating beyond words. He downplayed each of the symptoms which were playing havoc with my life. While he believed that nothing could be deduced from the "subjective complaint" of a pulsating feeling, he was at a loss to explain why the steroids had worked in the past. He conjectured that because I had worked in a doctor's office, I might be assuming the symptoms of patients with whom I had come in contact.

Vasculitis was ruled out because I had none of the identifying marks on my body. And although a disk problem in the lumbar area could be the cause of leg pain, it did not explain the pains in my arms.

The residents interjected at that point to remind him that I was unable to sleep through the night because of the pain. They asserted that I had provided a clear and complete history and that they found my story convincing. I consistently complained of pain in the same areas and of the same intensity.

The physician interrupted their comments on my behalf and asked them to review the medical information available. The blood results were almost consistently normal (they discounted a previously high ANA because it had been done at another institution); most other tests fell within normal limits. Nothing clinically significant had been found. He continued with the familiar words I had come to dread: In situations such as this, psychosomatic origins must be suspected.

The senior physician went on to explain that such patients typically have a long, well thought out story which incorporates a list of symptoms which can't be diagnosed. According to him, the best way to make the patient come to terms with the situation is to make her realize that she is not a "medical mystery" (as the residents had described me that morning). He suggested that the most helpful thing for them to do was tell me that I was perfectly healthy and that I had wasted a lot of time and money on unnecessary testing.

I cried so hard that I couldn't see the book in front of me. I wasn't particularly upset that one more doctor had refused to believe my story, but that I was no closer to a diagnosis, after all these new doctors, painful tests, and embarrassing exams. My translation of their conversation: No relief from the pain.

Discouraged beyond description, I called Eddie and told him what I had just heard. He had been through this with me before; his voice became even deeper and more sad. All I could feel was the unfairness of it all. I felt like someone accused of a crime I did not commit and unable to prove my innocence, when in fact I wasn't the criminal; I was the *victim*.

My fighting spirit was beginning to dissolve. The pain was just too severe to have to *justify* to these people. Yet, I could not explain why my test results were continually normal. I couldn't imagine what I would do next.

I had not come to any conclusions when Dr. Burke entered the room. I answered a few questions she had, and she recommended a pain clinic which she described as expensive but effective with patients having undiagnosed problems. I was glad that she never intimated that this was not an organic illness. Instead, she remained very realistic and suggested pain therapy as an interim step in what appeared to be a slow-moving disease. We would have to wait for more obvious symptoms to surface.

I asked her bluntly if she thought I had lupus. She believed that I did not, because none of the bloodwork indicated it. I watched her leave, impressed with her professionalism and dedication to helping me. I couldn't help but wonder whether she shared any of the skepticism I'd just overheard.

A third-year resident assigned to my case came in, and began a psychologically oriented interrogation. Was I under any particular stress at home? Was I looking forward to my daughter's return from camp? (An inane question, given that they saw the letters I sent to her daily.) How long had I been married? Was I a religious person? When he asked if I would consider seeing a psychiatrist while in the hospital, I simply said no. The two psychiatrists I had seen earlier recommended further *medical*, not psychological, evaluations.

He asked, in a sarcastic tone, if I wasn't being a little defensive, and I told him that I had already cooperated with that theory, and didn't intend to put any more time or money into something I knew was a deadend. I reminded him that anti-anxiety medication had had no effect on the pain. He had to admit that this did not support his psychological explanation.

I did not understand the doctors' confusion. It

seemed obvious to me that anxiety was not the cause of my problems. If anxiety troubled me, it had to do with the medical personnel's continual disbelief, and not with my loving and supportive family. I was being worn down by the people who were supposed to be helping me.

The string of visitors went on. The medical student came in, and I noticed the change in his attitude. Unlike the sincere, concerned person he had been earlier, he now acted absolutely pompous. Normally he pulled the curtain to provide some semblance of privacy as we talked. This time he left it wide open, although my roommate had visitors. Within earshot of everyone, he told me that I was a perfectly healthy thirty-five year old woman who had wasted a lot of time and money on unnecessary testing. I had to give him credit for having a good memory— he had memorized his supervisor's speech almost verbatim.

I decided to let him go on without informing him that I had already received that message. I made it clear that even though he advised against seeing any other physicians, I fully intended to do so. He argued, and I let his words fall on deaf ears.

8

Inner Changes, and a Significant Clue

As I rode home from the hospital, trying to concentrate despite an incredible headache, I realized again that what I needed was medical intervention and scrutiny by *one* coordinating physician. In spite of the many specialists involved, I still carried the burden of being the one to suggest ideas, ask about tests, and question possible diagnoses. I felt overwhelmed with all this responsibility, and I needed the *doctors* to take control so that I could use all my energy for recovering.

I continued to argue with myself: Was I being unrealistic? The doctors didn't know what they were dealing with. Was I impatient? I kept pursuing theories because I was the one in daily, uninterrupted pain. I didn't know how much longer I could stand it.

When I contacted Dr. Dupont the next day, I was surprised to learn that no one from the hospital had been in touch with him. This only validated my decision to find one physician who would handle the many details of my case. I told Dr. Dupont about the latest trials at the hospital, and let him know that I did not feel qualified, able, or willing to continue to coordinate my complicated health care.

I had already decided against a pain therapy program; it turned out to be even more expensive than I had expected. Instead, I suggested that we try steroid therapy again, the only treatment that had any effect on the pain. Could I take a higher, and hopefully more effective, dosage this time? Dr. Dupont agreed, with the qualification that no matter how much the steroids helped me, I was only to use them for a two-month trial period. There were too many potentially harmful side effects for him to promise me more than this. I was glad to agree to his limits.

Within five days on the steroid medication, I was sleeping through the night. I'd say my level of pain was cut by a third. It was working! The numbness and pulsations continued, but whatever I had was being attacked and threatened. Doubling the steroid dose brought even more improvement. Walking, driving, and simply standing, which had become monumental undertakings, became much easier.

I was filled with optimism, which was undoubtedly premature. Even with the significant decrease in pain, I was still extremely uncomfortable. The medication also added to my fatigue, and I began to take naps throughout the day.

Both my increasing fatigue and the fact that I was helped so much by steroids, which are commonly used to treat connective tissue diseases, might have been solid clues toward a diagnosis. But in themselves, these were not conclusive evidence. It took one very visible outbreak to pull all of the threads together.

As I washed my face one morning, I noticed a bumpy, symmetrical rash on my cheeks. When it did not go away, I called Dr. Dupont. Here at last was a "clinically significant" sign. He was certain that I would have been diagnosed with lupus if this rash had erupted during my hospitalization.

Did this prove, finally, that I had lupus? He referred to it as a "piece of the puzzle." For someone who had been through what I had, that wasn't good enough! I didn't want to hear about puzzle pieces—I wanted answers!

I was tired of being told to be patient. I had been patient from the onset—through surgeries, biopsies, tests, examinations, doctors who wouldn't return my calls, and humiliating psychological interrogations. I knew that I had been far more patient than was good for me. I confided to Sue, who had come by for a visit, that while I had been hopeful all these months that I had something curable, I was beginning to think that this was overly idealistic.

While we sat together, entertaining the discouraging possibility that what I had would be with me forever, the phone rang. It was the rheumatologist from the hospital, who had been so thoughtful. Dr. Burke's tone was more serious than I remembered as she related my final test results. To my overwhelming relief, MS had been conclusively eliminated as a possibility.

She had interesting news about the muscle biopsy which had been done in conjunction with the sural nerve procedure. Although a normal report had been sent back to her, and her clinic's reevaluation had also come out normal, the peculiarity of my pain had made her suspicious. She consulted a neuromuscular pathologist for yet another opinion, and this doctor disagreed with the earlier evaluations. The pathologist felt that this was one of the most abnormal biopsies she had ever seen. She was not able to determine what the abnormality signified, and wanted another biopsy ordered immediately, using a different staining technique.

I was not at all surprised that something had finally been found, and I was *angry*. This was the same hospital which had so rudely told me that there was no clinical evidence for my illness. Granted, Dr. Burke was not the one who had passed this judgment, but why hadn't she consulted with the other doctors? I told her that I would have to talk with my own doctor and my family before going ahead with another biopsy.

As I thought about all that I had been through, I found myself overwhelmed with empathy for the hundreds or possibly thousands of people like me, also in terrible pain, but lacking clinical evidence to substantiate it. How many others have gone through months of expense and aggravation to reach a diagnosis? Perhaps this problem was typical; what a terrifying thought. I knew then that I needed to describe my experience for others. If I could offer a patient's point of view of an undiagnosed illness, perhaps it would spare even a few people the trauma I had been through.

In order to have the second biopsy, I would have to discontinue the steroid treatment. I was very reluctant to stop, since it was my only source of pain relief. Dr. Dupont agreed with me that the muscle biopsy could wait until we had finished this trial period. If it still seemed necessary, a biopsy could be performed then.

Dr. Dupont had a long conversation with Dr. Burke, who stated clearly that this was not a psychosomatic illness. I was grateful for that concession, but concerned as to how long she would continue to feel that way without further clinical substantiation. Would I be put to another test? I hated to see this bitter attitude surface, although I certainly thought it was understandable.

Dr. Dupont and I discussed the emotional drain which accompanies the long wait for a diagnosis. I had to admit that the hardest part for me, in addition to the physical manifestations, was trying to convince everyone that I was sick. As I reflect back on our conversation, I see that what I did *not* verbalize was how very frightened I was. We had no conclusive diagnosis, my entire body was affected, and the symptoms only got worse. Even with the prescribed dosage of steroids, I had some very difficult days. At times I could not sit at the table and reach out for my spoon or fork without bursting into tears.

Although I had become more realistic about my limitations, I was still uncomfortable accepting help, even from Eddie. I was a prime example of denial, attending parties and lunches that I sat through in absolute misery. I tried to wish the illness away or forget about it. I don't know who I was trying to fool with this conviction that I could maintain my normal lifestyle.

As disconcerting as this is for me to admit, I was embarrassed by the physical debilitation that was obvious to everyone. A whole new range of emotions opened up for me. On the positive side, I was becoming more sensitive to people with handicaps of any kind; on the other hand, I was opposed to accepting help, convinced that it would be a step backward, making me more dependent.

I can recall a disturbing incident at a woman's club dinner which I attended with Sue. I had trouble cutting my meat because of the pain in my upper arms and shoulders. Sue offered to help. Although I would have felt comfortable having her do this in private, I was too self-conscious to accept her help in front of everyone else. What a foolish decision! I wonder now if others in this situation have the same trouble with pride. I can see now that this is an area in which a therapist can be of great help.

My slowly changing attitude made it easier to tolerate some of my limitations. When I sensed that something was beyond my physical abilities, I admitted it. If uncomfortable sitting, I would elevate my legs, even out in public. I began to cancel commitments, even when it hurt my pride to do so. Openly acknowledging some of my limitations allowed others to be more honest with me. Accepting the facts of my illness was much easier than trying to keep up what was clearly an absurd front.

It was the middle of October and I had been on steroids for about a month and a half. The improvement, unfortunately, was not remarkable. Other tasks began to be difficult: rolling up the car window, dressing, standing in the shower. I began to feel that no matter how hard I tried, I was losing the battle. In many instances, I no longer had a choice whether or not to do something; my body made the decision for me.

The pain began to increase again. I overheard with envy the peaceful, rhythmic sounds of my family sleeping, as I watched darkness change to daylight night after night. Trying to distract myself from the pain, I spent many of my nights writing the first drafts of this book. Eddie would wake in the morning to find me with red, stinging eyes, dizzy from lack of sleep.

At my next appointment with Dr. Dupont, I described exactly what I was experiencing. Even though

I continued to have the butterfly rash, all lupus-related bloodwork came back negative. We talked in detail about muscle-related diseases, and the degree of my muscle weakness.

I told him that I was just plain frustrated with myself, lying awake night after night wondering why I could not describe my symptoms so that some conclusions could be drawn. He reassured me that I had always been very clear in my descriptions; the length of time that it was taking to reach a diagnosis had nothing to do with any lack of effort on my part.

My arms and back were noticeably more sensitive than they had been, as he gently examined my muscles. The slightest touch was uncomfortable. The pain was not diminishing as we had hoped it would through the steroid treatment, and we decided to discontinue it. He told me to increase the dosage of my pain medication to counteract the discomfort which would appear as the steroids left my system. And he promised to contact a hospital which specialized in collagen diseases (collagen being the primary substance in connective tissue and bones). I went home confident that at least now something was being done; we were testing our options, and would eventually discover one that worked.

Despite the perfect sleeping weather of a cool October evening, I was wide awake, occupied with discouraging thoughts. I couldn't sleep even on a sizable steroid dosage (40 mg. per day, at this point). What did this say about the severity of my illness? I had been told that diseases such as the ones I was suspected of having were often brought under control by 5 mg. per day! I had to face the fact that my condition was getting worse.

With a weekend in Vermont up and coming, I was worried. But I wasn't about to let anything prevent me from going. Eddie and I had selected a quiet country inn, which sounded perfect.

This turned out to be, by far, the most special weekend away that we had ever shared. The inn was furnished in authentic colonial style, and had been constructed in 1803. The rooms were spacious and comfortable, with hand-stenciled patterns on the walls. It was a small place, which made for genuine conversations among the guests. The innkeepers were more than accommodating, and the food surpassed that of the best restaurants I have visited.

This place suited us perfectly. We had long talks and leisurely dinners. We took a back country ride to several colonial college towns, sipped hot spiced cider at an old-fashioned soda parlor, sang our favorite songs, and relaxed.

We also—unfortunately, inevitably—worried. Eddie and I talked for hours about my health. Although I had pain medication with me, the steroids had by then been reduced by 25% and I noticed it. The pulsating feeling had returned throughout my body, the numbness was more prominent, and the muscle pain and burning increased. The cozy patchwork quilt provided at the inn was too heavy for my sensitive muscles. I could not sleep at all the first night, but I functioned well enough to enjoy the next day, having become accustomed to little sleep. I scheduled the pain medication strategically, saving it until I could no longer wait, and reserving it for special activities. By Saturday evening, the pain was so intense that I didn't know what else to try; I had used everything in my bag of tricks.

I was equally upset for Eddie, who told me how much it hurt him to see me in pain. He likened my illness to a tap of running water. He saw the pain as the constant flow of water, but the tap had no handle for him to control or alleviate the flow. Though there were times when he could help by massaging a sore muscle, at other times he knew that just a touch brought intense pain. With tear-filled eyes, he described his feelings when he awoke in the middle of the night to the sounds of my sobs of pain.

What a difficult year it had been for him. I tried to imagine *him* having the illness, and me sitting back, forced to watch him suffer. I immediately tried to destroy the depressing picture that thought conjured up in my mind.

In spite of our sadness, we agreed, as we packed on our last morning at the inn, that this had been an important time together. Over breakfast at a roadside diner, headed home, we promised to return to the inn together the next year. It was a hopeful, loving vow to make in an uncertain time.

9

The First Year Draws to a Close

During the first weeks of November, as the effects of the steroid medication decreased, my pain level steadily increased. I found myself becoming more and more apprehensive about the holidays.

We were planning to celebrate Thanksgiving with relatives who lived nearby, a tradition which meant a lot to all of us. I questioned the logic of leaving home, given how I felt, but decided to go for our family's sake. Once again, I had made the wrong decision. Before dinner was over, I had to leave the table. Taking more medication and putting my legs up was not enough, and we left for home after only a few hours together.

When I had been off the steroids long enough to clear my system, Dr. Dupont ran more blood tests. There were still no signs that would point to a diagnosis.

December is one of my favorite months. I have always gone into the holidays full of excitement and anticipation, but this year I was extremely depressed. I knew very well that I was nearing the one-year mark: a full year of incapacitating illness which dozens of doctors were at a loss to explain.

Even the small pleasures of the season became losses. I love selecting special gifts for a long list of friends and family. I was used to planning and shopping all on my own. Now I had to go out more often, for very short periods. Because I couldn't drive far by myself, there were few places I could shop independent of Eddie or my friends.

When the time approached for the Christmas party at Dr. Dupont's office, I sat down and reflected on my situation. Last year I had played a part in all the festivities. I did not want to give up every holiday activity, and at the same time I knew that there was nothing more I could do to normalize my life. Why couldn't this be a bad dream? Wasn't there some magic which would take me back to December of 1983, when I had such a simple and happy life?

I called Dr. Dupont to say that the pain was becoming worse, and we reviewed our options. After carefully weighing the alternatives, we agreed to Dr. Burke's earlier suggestion: I would return to the teaching hospital for another muscle biopsy. Dr. Burke and the neuromuscular pathologist who had evaluated my first biopsy as abnormal would review the new results.

I went to meet the surgeon in early December, and showed him the muscle area where I had the most consistent pain, on my right thigh. He assured me that I would be able to mark the spot myself before surgery, and he would use that as his incision point. He allayed my fear that a resident might be doing the procedure; I wanted his experience behind this operation, since I had had so much work done already with so little result. He gave me his word that he would be doing the surgery, and I felt greatly relieved. Happily, we were able to forego the two-week wait for an appointment, which would have had me in surgery during the holiday. We were called in on a cancellation; Eddie and I left the house at 5:30 in the morning to meet the early surgery schedule. I discussed with the anesthesiologist the type of medication he and my surgeon believed would be most appropriate. Because I had been on steroids so recently, the surgeon preferred that I remain awake. They decided to use a nerve-blocking technique, which could be supplemented with shots if necessary. I would also be given something to relax me. This combination had proved effective in surgeries more major than the one I was about to undergo.

I began to shake as I was wheeled into the operating room. My surgeon asked, in a kind voice, if I was afraid of the surgery. No, I was not worried that I was about to have surgery. I was shaking because this was my third surgery for the same disease, and I wanted it to be the last. I knew there were no guarantees, but I needed and wanted an answer.

The procedure turned out to be absolutely interesting. I was completely coherent for the hour it took to complete, aware of everything that was said and done. The surgeon had asked me to tell him if he reached a particularly sensitive area, and, when I did, he injected a numbing medication there. Although I could not see the actual operation because of a screen in front of me, the surgeon explained when he reached the outermost part of the muscle, when he was going deeper, and when he was about to close the incision. We talked about the sensations I felt, and the anesthesiologist stayed at my side answering my questions. I listened to what was said to an observing resident. How completely different this was from my earlier operations. I felt like a respected participant in my own care.

As I talked with Eddie in the recovery room, a nurse noticed the pink, raised rash on my face—the "butterfly" presentation. Eddie and I had thought nothing of it; I had had this rash every day for several months—symmetrical marks across my cheeks, with a little connecting section across my nose.

The nurse called Dr. Burke, who was at my bedside within minutes. I was let down at her inability to make a diagnosis given all the evidence she now had, but she cautioned me that it would be more damaging to be misdiagnosed. Also, she felt I should not put too much hope in the results of the muscle biopsy. It could come back normal, or, even if it showed abnormalities, the doctors might not know what to make of it.

I was even more discouraged when she told me that, in some situations, very little can be done; I might have to "learn to live with it." As I considered this pain going on and on, I began to cry. Dr. Burke said that she would call in a week with the results of the biopsy and blood tests. I had to thank her as she left; I knew she was doing her best, and she was infinitely more sensitive than many of the doctors I'd seen.

That night in bed, I prayed that something definitive would come out of these tests. I did not know how much longer I could go on without some kind of treatment. Although I had no reason to expect the blood tests to show anything, I was hoping that something might be uncovered because I had selected the most painful spot on my body for the biopsy. It would be another long week of waiting.

About a week before Christmas, Stacey and Storey decorated our Christmas tree. This was the first year I did not take part. Although it was a sad occasion for me, I was grateful that they were old enough to handle it themselves. They did a wonderful job—the tree was beautiful, and we sang carols and sipped hot chocolate in front of the fire when it was finished.

The children's Christmas party at the Jaycees took place the next day. Stacey and Storey prepared their lists for Santa, full of excitement. I stayed in bed the entire day, trying to gather enough energy so that I could go, but when the time came I knew that I could not make it through the evening. Although the incision ached, what prevented me from going was my overall pain.

I looked at Storey, dressed up and eager, and realized that this might be the last Christmas that she believed in Santa Claus. The holidays were full of milestones and markers, and it was so difficult not to be part of them.

I tried to leave the phone free throughout the week, though I knew that the results would not be ready until Friday. Each day that I did not receive a call, I worried. Maybe nothing would show up. Maybe everything would come out normal again, and they would want to refer me to another psychiatrist. How would I react if they went that route again? I continued to pray.

When Friday afternoon came, and I still had heard nothing, I called Dr. Burke. I expected to hear that everything was normal. If anything had shown up that was *abnormal*, they certainly would have called before this. And yet, it seemed impossible that the biopsy could be normal, given the constant pain in the area of the muscle sample.

To my complete surprise, Dr. Burke explained that the delay in contacting me was because the muscle slides definitely *were* abnormal and, furthermore, were not easily related to a particular disease. She had spent several days showing the slides to specialists at the hospital. They could see an obvious muscle abnormality, but none of them could identify the source. They now knew the parts of the body affected by the disease, and needed to evaluate further to find a way to treat the symptoms.

As she was expressing regret that she could not give me an exact diagnosis, I interrupted her: She had no idea how *relieved* I was that she had a clinically significant finding. This was more than I had been given in an entire year! Our next step would be an appointment with a muscle specialist, which she hoped to arrange within the next two weeks.

I called Dr. Dupont to relay the good news. He felt comfortable with the course of action and, although wanting to be reassuring, was also noncommittal. We were still dealing with so many different possible diagnoses that he wanted neither to paint a pessimistic picture nor give me false hope.

He asked if I was discouraged. Actually, I said, I was very encouraged. Now, at last, we had something to work with.

That night, unable to sleep even with pain medication, I could only lie in bed and think. The more I thought, the more apprehensive I became. I knew I had a problem with my muscles. I did not know if it could be treated or how serious it was. The pain ran throughout my entire body, and any exertion exhausted me. Once again, I worried about the possibility of paralysis. I found myself trying to move my legs as soon as I woke up each morning, just to be sure I could. I was scared.

On Christmas Eve, we traditionally have our relatives over for a big dinner. I hoped that, with careful planning and some major modifications, we could pull it off, so that the year would not be a complete exception to our regular family life. I did far less than in other years, and the evening was great fun. Still, I was completely drained. After church on Christmas day, I went right to bed. Eddie and the girls had dinner with the relatives, though they did not want to leave me alone. I was happy to be able to sleep.

The pain continued to increase. I stayed in touch with Dr. Burke, who was still circulating the slides of the muscle biopsy among various specialists. Though they could identify a problem in the muscles, they could not give it a name. We scheduled an appointment for March with a muscle specialist, and concluded that we would proceed on the basis of his advice.

As New Year's Eve approached, I was in a real dilemma about what to do. I considered having dinner at our home with a few good friends, rather than attending the town dance. Did I really want to spend the evening sitting out all of my favorite songs? Yet, this night had become a wonderful tradition. We would be with so many close friends. It would not be the same without them, and the laughter, and the music. Eddie and I decided that we simply had to go.

Most of our usual group of old friends was there—including Sue, Jen, Keith, and Denise. Others we had recently come to know joined us. It helped my spirits to hear so many people say that this was going to be a better year. As I sat, enjoying the color and movement of the crowd, I thought about last year's party, here at the same hall. I was so healthy then. How dramatically life had changed. I wondered how I would feel at this time *next* year.

I confided these fears to some of my closest friends, and, rather than tell me that I should stop worrying, they simply listened. It was what I needed most. I had a terrific time, but my anxiety was still with me as I crawled into bed on the first morning of a new year.

10

A Diagnosis
At Last

It was brisk on the morning I was to be admitted for tests with the muscle specialist. The air threatened snow. Saying good-bye to Stacey and Storey was always difficult, particularly when I did not know how long I would be away from them. But the deep muscle pain which had kept me awake all night convinced me that this trip was for *everyone's* benefit. My increasing immobility and absence from family activities was a drain on us all. We hoped that this hospitalization would lead to a diagnosis, so we could get on with our life as a family.

Over a quiet lunch, breaking up the long ride to the hospital in Massachusetts, Eddie and I shared our concerns and hopes about this latest effort. What we wanted most was a treatment program which would reduce my excruciating pain. Though experience had cautioned us about being too optimistic, we were both impressed by the myologist's reputation and how he had handled my case thus far. He had been sent my medical history and the biopsy slides.

In a phone consultation, we discussed his initial evaluation: This might be a glycogen storage disease, late-onset muscular dystrophy, or a connective tissue disease such as lupus.

Eddie and I discussed every possibility, and his eyes reflected my own hope and fear. His support meant everything to me. When I woke up in tears, night after night, his voice reassured me in the dark. No matter how late it was, or how early he had to be up for work the next morning, he always made time to talk with me and to listen. He would reach out to hold me, and I would have to move away; the weight of even his touch was more than my muscles could tolerate. Sadly, on many nights, even a gentle hug, which we both wanted so much, was impossible. Sometimes, when I was able to fall asleep, he would touch my hand, and it caused enough pain to wake me up. My heart ached thinking how much our situation needed to change.

We arrived at the medical center shortly after noon. I sighed with relief as the receptionist found my name on her inpatient admission list; I always had the momentary fear that we had come on the wrong day. I settled down next to Eddie on one of the leather couches. Its soft give was soothing after two hours in the car. The hospital was impressive: marble floors, a cathedral ceiling in the lobby, the smell of leather, sculptured columns around the walls of the waiting room.

I was reminded of the administration building of the college I had attended more than ten years before. How carefree my life had been then. Coping with this illness would have been easier with only myself to be concerned about. At least all of my energies could be invested in one direction—getting well. Instead, I was worried not only about myself but about Eddie and the girls. Rather than concentrating on what was taking place at this hospital, I was mentally listing the things I had forgotten to do at home—mail that needed to be answered, dental appointments to be made.

More important, I was worrying about the effect of all my absences on Stacey and Storey, and about the unspoken fears they surely had about my continuing presence in their lives. Even the way I handled my illness had to be different because I was a mother. I cannot count the times I attempted to cover up my anxiety when I knew how important some event was for the girls, or how often I wiped tears of pain from my eyes and put on a big, reassuring smile if they awoke at night and came running into the bedroom. Clearly, being a wife, mother, and patient all at once was overwhelming.

Eddie came with me for my preliminary blood-work, X-rays, and an electrocardiogram. When all the tests were completed, we were escorted to my room. Even the stark metal bed looked inviting after the long car ride and the extended admission procedures. This was far more activity than I had in a regular day. I changed quickly and unpacked, looking forward to an hour or two with Eddie. But as we settled in, we could see outside the beginnings of a storm; if Eddie wanted to make the long ride home safely, he would have to leave immediately.

A resident came in just then to examine me, and I quickly kissed Eddie and reminded him to drive carefully. Even our brief good-bye communicated an underlying message that much could happen before we saw each other again. Eddie promised to call when he got home.

As I watched him walk out the door, I resisted my urge to call him back and ask him to stay and hold me. I was terrified about my undecided future. Maybe I could book a room for him locally, and let the kids stay with friends or relatives. No, Stacey and Storey needed him as much as I did. I bit my tongue to silence the suggestion before it got to my lips, and hoped that this was not another decision I would come to regret.

The resident's questioning distracted me from my worries. She shook her head in disbelief throughout the detailed story of my surgeries and misdiagnoses. She assured me that, if I could wait for another week or so, I would be feeling much more comfortable than I had since the onset of the disease.

This seemed too good to be true. I was still undiagnosed, after all the promises. I had been told the back surgery would cure my problems; when it did not, I was told that the first teaching hospital was the place to go. Why should I believe this person? Still, she was appalled by my medical history and genuinely interested in my current symptoms, and I clung to her encouraging words. I needed her to be right.

I had to warn her that any bloodwork she ordered would probably come out normal, and was glad to see that the comment did not take the confident look from her eyes. I tried to guard my enthusiasm as she left the room, and later, when I talked to Eddie, I think I conveyed some very mixed feelings.

Considering that I had seen more hospitals than I cared to remember, I settled into the routine in this latest institution as best I could. I was particularly grateful for the nurses. They were obviously accustomed to treating people isolated from their family and friends, and although I missed Eddie and the girls, I will always be grateful to the staff on my floor for helping to compensate for the loneliness. On that first night, as I lay awake in pain, caring nurses sat on my bed and reassured me. They had seen many patients with rare diseases which were finally diagnosed at this hospital, even when other specialists had been thoroughly baffled. They spoke highly of my physician and told me success stories. They offered hot and cold packs, pain medication, and company through the long night. Though none of their ministrations could take away my pain, the support was a welcome change from my previous hospitalizations.

While eating a big breakfast the next morning, I was taken off-guard by my doctor coming through the door with a group so large that everyone could not get into the room at the same time. I shrank back into the bed; I was much more comfortable in one-to-one medical encounters. The doctor initiated a dialogue with me which allowed him to instruct the group about my curious disease.

One thing was clear from the teaching session: I knew the characteristics of this illness. I identified when, where, and how I hurt and distinguished the various types of pain I experienced. Unlike other patients who I'd heard say "pain is pain," I knew there were different ways to describe it, because I felt it at such different levels. I detailed the deep, penetrating muscle pain, as opposed to the intense, burning pain on the surface of my skin. I named the specific joints which ached routinely, and I pointed out that my tendons also hurt relentlessly, causing me as much pain at rest as during activity. I mentioned my transient blurry vision and excessive hair loss. It seemed superfluous to mention the bright red rash which ran across my cheeks and nose.

Thinking about the rash reminded me how obsessed I had become with pointing out "clinical evidence," after having heard so often that there *was* none. As in my previous hospitalizations, I felt compelled to call in a nurse to document each occurrence of the rash, until a resident responded to one of my calls and let me know that this was unnecessary—everyone *believed* me. I realized that I desperately feared being told again that there was nothing wrong. I almost expected to be sent home again without any way to control the pain.

Shortly after the crowd left the room, I heard rolling rubber wheels against the tile floor as an orderly came to take me to the EMG area for muscle testing. The doctor there helped me out of the wheelchair, and I explained to him that I had recently had these tests performed in my home state, with normal results. This doctor, who I recognized as one of the people who had come in on rounds that morning, explained that his procedure was slightly different, taking into account the abnormalities which had shown up on the muscle biopsy.

His test *was* different. Although he used needles to measure muscle activity in the same areas, the test was administered at a deeper level, which caused me more pain. Watching the results on a screen, he indicated that there definitely were abnormalities appearing. I broke out in a cold sweat, remembering how relieved my family doctor had been when my earlier EMG had been normal. Had this doctor discovered one of the more severe muscle diseases? I was taken back to my room briefly, then the same orderly appeared again to transport me to the operating room for the muscle biopsy.

By this point, I was overcome with exhaustion. It had been a draining, endless morning, and surgery was well behind schedule. I waited in the wheelchair for an hour, until my muscles became too weak to hold me in a sitting position. I asked if I could lie down, and was immediately put into a bed and left to rest for another hour.

A surgeon finally appeared, explaining that he planned to make a three-inch incision in my left shin to obtain the muscle tissue. I remembered how I had worried about scarring with the first biopsy; it couldn't be further from my mind now. It was one hour, without complications, from the local anesthetic being administered to the doctor's announcement that the procedure was over.

For the rest of the week I had extensive blood-work done and biopsies of my constant facial rash. My face, neck, and stomach were now turning bright purple-red, deeper than a severe sunburn. In a way, I was relieved; these rashes were supposed to be meaningful, and might help the process move along more quickly.

On Friday, my doctor informed me that they had conducted most of the tests they needed. Although some results were still outstanding, he planned to begin a regimen of high dosage steroids the next week. He wanted me hospitalized during the beginning of the treatment, so that my condition would be monitored while I was on the high level of prednisone. (Prednisone, while offering relief to many people with different illnesses, has a long list of serious side effects. It is only cautiously prescribed for long-term use.)

Since no testing would be done over the weekend, I was given a 48-hour break to return home. When most people leave a hospital, they want it to be for good; I was no exception. I did not like the idea of returning on Monday.

When Eddie appeared in my room on Saturday morning, he had never looked so good. Getting dressed that morning had been such an effort that I was lying down again when he arrived. The resident stopped by, took one look at me, and asked if I was sure I wanted to go home. Though I knew I felt terrible, I missed my family, and talking on the phone only made me more anxious to see them. I chose to ignore the resident's concern and my own intuition. The ride home worsened my fatigue, though I had loaded up on pain medication. Eddie was so worried about me that he wanted to go back that afternoon. I decided to wait out the weekend, rationalizing that I would get no help until Monday anyway, when the order for steroids went into effect.

It was the most painful period I had had since the illness began. Virtually useless to my family, and having to admit to myself that the disease was progressing at an alarming pace, I found myself counting the hours until I could return to the hospital. I was back in bed there in time for Monday morning rounds.

At midday, the resident appeared with a medical student to conduct more bloodwork. The resident had to poke me repeatedly and apologized profusely. I did not care how many jabs it took, if it meant learning something about my situation. It did not seem fair, she said, that I had had such a difficult year, when my medical history showed so many abnormalities. As she touched my hand, I was again reminded of the empathy and concern I had finally found at this hospital.

That night, it took only a walk of a few yards to the nurses' station to bring me to tears. No amount of pain medication helped. I was afraid to think about what could be wrong with me, and I knew I was on the verge of finding out.

Tuesday morning I was given my first dose of prednisone. After taking 20 mg. three times a day for three days, my pain decreased noticeably. I was ecstatic. By the fourth day, the pain was cut nearly in half. Even more important, I was sleeping through the night and able to stand for longer periods. My rashes faded, returning only when I was due for another dose of prednisone.

Though I had prayed for a diagnosis all these months, I was unprepared emotionally when it finally came. On Friday morning rounds, my doctor informed me that, based on all the clinical evidence and my response to the steroids, I had an inflammatory connective tissue disease.

I was speechless for several moments. After this long battle, a doctor finally knew what was wrong and was doing something which would help me. After all the times I had been told that I was wasting time and money, that I should get psychological help. . . . I began angrily to make a mental list of the ridiculous reasons other physicians had offered for my symptoms: too much coffee, masturbation anxiety, hyperventilation—even voodoo was suggested! I remembered one doctor telling me that I was not to come back to him until a psychiatrist had "cured" me, and the one who repeatedly insisted that my symptoms did not make "good medical sense." All the mixed emotions which had built up inside me over the past year began to run rampant. I was relieved, angry, and frightened at the same time.

Unfortunately, the myologist still had to wait for final test results before he could provide answers to the barrage of questions I threw at him. He finally convinced me that I would have to settle for this preliminary diagnosis. I managed to learn two important things from him: the name of my illness and that he did not believe this would be either paralyzing or fatal. After more than a year of worrying. . . I cannot begin to describe the freedom and relief I felt at that moment.

I was released with a prescription for steroids and anti-inflammatory medication, and we scheduled a follow-up appointment in one month. Eddie and I were bursting with relief; we talked all the way home. Although I knew, given this diagnosis, that my life would not be easy, I was sure now that I could get through whatever happened.

One of my first steps was to contact the Lupus Foundation and explain my recent diagnosis. Although I had not specifically been diagnosed with lupus, it was a real possibility. The people I spoke with were very encouraging, and knew exactly what I was talking about. They invited us to their next meeting, where we were greeted with a wealth of information and the kind of knowing, caring support we had been seeking from the beginning.

My symptoms, though they were reduced by the steroid treatment, were constant and fatiguing. It was clear that this was not going to be easy to live with, but we had made a start. I had a name for my pain, and a community of people who understood.

11

Moving On

Throughout April I responded well to the steroid treatment. The high dosage allowed me a much more normal life-style. I was able to stand for longer periods and could do more with Stacey and Storey. Social events were infinitely easier. We were able as a family to enjoy a week on Cape Cod at the end of the month. This time was especially pleasurable, after so many ruined vacations. Even though I was still extremely fatigued and weak, and had developed other symptoms, including ulcers in my mouth and nose, we all felt tremendously optimistic. I was sure that I had finally turned the corner with this illness.

When we arrived home after the three and a half hour ride from the Cape, I thought nothing of a slight cramp in my left leg. I'd been sitting a long time, and everything was going so well. Over the course of that week, I would occasionally wake up with that same cramp—not severe, but sharp enough to bother me. The calf muscle continued to tighten as the days went by. Unlike my other muscle tightness, which could be relieved with heat, massage, or moisture, this was unresponsive.

I had a midweek appointment with Dr. Michaels, my rheumatologist. I was anxious to hear his response to the latest findings from the teaching hospital. He told me that while I did have a connective tissue disease, it was not one of the simple inflammatory types. I had systemic lupus erythematosus—I had lupus. In a more serious and direct manner than I could remember him using before, he explained that this was a disease for which there was currently no cure. I was frightened by the pessimistic prognosis, but, at the same time, grateful that he was leveling with me.

Considering that the steroid treatment had seemed less effective over the last weeks, even at the high dosage, the more serious diagnosis didn't really surprise me. I decided that Dr. Michaels should act as my primary physician, since lupus is clearly a rheumatological problem.

As the week went on, my leg worsened to the point that I needed a cane to walk, and people on the street began to offer me assistance. I remember telling a friend that if I were in the path of an oncoming car, I wouldn't be able to move out of the way.

On Saturday we went to a large outdoor party at the home of friends. I was practically immobile all day and in intense pain again. Storey fell down while playing and cut her lip, and I could not even stand up to help her. I did not feel like much of a mother as I watched Eddie and a friend comfort her.

Just before midnight that evening, my left leg swelled to twice its normal size. I was reluctant to call Dr. Michaels in the middle of the night, and felt even less sure when I did call and was put through to my doctor's partner, whom I had never met. When I explained to him that I was a lupus patient and described the swelling, he suspected I had phlebitis, which requires immediate treatment. He called the emergency room to alert them of our arrival, and we woke the children and got into the car.

The doctor in ER agreed that this was a classic case of phlebitis, which in my condition was dangerous. I was given a blood-thinner and put on continual bedrest. At about 1:30 in the morning, after a nurse had given the girls some crackers and juice, we said our good-byes.

Storey was especially disappointed by all the confusion, because it meant that we could not keep our anniversary breakfast date that morning. On the morning that we first met Storey at the airport, after the long months of adoption proceedings, we excitedly claimed her and immediately went out for a celebratory breakfast as a new family. Every year since, we had gone out for breakfast on that day to remember the special event she is in our lives. I promised her that we would have our meal together as soon as I was able to come home.

I had constant care throughout the night. My vital signs were monitored closely, moist heat was applied to my leg, and I received medication intravenously. Dr. Michael's partner came in the next morning on rounds. Any apprehension I had about seeing a new physician was dissolved by his concerted effort to put me at ease. He made it clear that coming in to the hospital was not only the right move, but an essential one. They suspected that a blood clot had caused the swelling. When left untreated, a blood clot can travel within the circulatory system—in the worst case, causing a stroke if it enters the heart. I would remain on the blood thinner until Monday, when a venogram would be done. The results of this test, in which dye is injected into a vein in the foot, would verify the presence of phlebitis and determine the extent of its damage.

I talked with Eddie about my great sense of relief now that my doctors knew what I had, how to treat it, and that it could be controlled. With this peace of mind, I was ready to have the venogram done. It proved to be an uneventful procedure.

I gave in to a long overdue nap, as anyone could see I needed by the dark circles shadowing my eyes. I was startled out of a dream by my friend Diane. We had lost touch after that painful day at her house when she, too, had questioned the validity of my illness. Though so much had happened during our silence, we hugged, and I knew nothing had really changed between us.

Diane sadly explained how much other friends' opinions had influenced her. I had realized that long ago, but it was reassuring to hear her say it. The close feelings between us returned without any struggle. How I had missed her company! Her visit was one of the most healing gifts I could have received.

Dr. Michaels came in the next day with the results of the venogram, and I couldn't believe what I was hearing. The results were completely negative. I did not have phlebitis. They would not be able to tell me what the problem was until they had done "further testing"—a phrase I had come to hate.

The blood-thinning medication and bed rest were discontinued. But when I was allowed up on my feet even for a few seconds, my leg swelled and immediately turned dark purple. I remained in the hospital for almost three weeks, undergoing tests and minor diagnostic surgical procedures.

By the time I was released, both Dr. Michaels and I were completely frustrated. The conclusion, after all the tests, was that I had had a flare-up of lupus-related inflammation and muscle weakness. Whether

it would travel to my other limbs could not be
predicted. All I knew was that I was leaving the hospital in many ways worse off than when I had come in.

I could not believe it—I had suddenly become
handicapped. I needed a walker and what seemed an
incredible array of special equipment, not to mention
the services of visiting nurses and physical therapists.
All of this was new to me. I could not drive and,
initially, I was instructed to stay off my leg in the
hopes that it would simply heal by itself. Walking up
stairs was impossible, and I had to get off the couch
on all fours.

I remembered the teaching hospital's physician
telling me not to worry about losing my ability to
walk. This was not supposed to happen, and I did not
handle it well. Using the walker embarrassed me, and
I resented needing others to prepare meals and transport my children. If I had not been so stubbornly
independent before, this latest turn might have been
easier for me to handle. Although I was accustomed
to volunteering and helping others in my town, I was
just not ready to accept help for myself.

Fortunately, I had a number of good friends, even
given the strain on many of the friendships. They all
seemed to come forward during this bout. The nurses
described my room as a "gift shop," with its floor to
ceiling balloons, posters, flowers, cards, and stuffed
animals. One of my visitors aptly called it a room full
of love. The same friends who had decorated my room
came through in other ways. I saw their real concern
reflected in every visit, as they listened to my worries
and needs. I know that their love and support, along
with that of my family, is what allowed me to make
the difficult adjustment from the hospital to my home.

At first I was scared when I realized what a false
sense of security the hospital had provided. I no

longer had bed rails, call buttons, special bathroom facilities, and 24-hour medical care. But I did have the emotional and practical support of my family, friends, and doctor. Gradually, and with much encouragement, I began to adjust. Although I was not immediately ready to face the general public, I found that sharing time with my close friends made things easier. With their acceptance, I became less self-conscious.

Perhaps the most difficult "test" I attempted was when our dinner club met at the home of good friends a few blocks away. Everyone attending was part of a close circle. It was my first attempt at socializing since the hospitalization, and I knew it would not be easy. I was going to have to accept help in front of everyone. I knew I could not handle the steps leading into the house without assistance, and I would not be able to get up from any of the easy chairs. I hesitated, but everyone encouraged me to come.

I was glad I listened to the encouragement of these people whose opinions I valued. They had anticipated all my needs and had made the house ready so that the evening was as comfortable as if I had been in my own home. The seating was arranged around my comfort and, most important, the room was full of caring friends who did not ask questions or judge. I needed that evening so badly, and loved them all for it. Their confidence made me want to try harder.

That one night gave me the impetus to go out on other occasions. Though I was still self-conscious, I learned that it is healthier to swallow a little pride— or in my case, a lot!—than to sit at home. Gradually, I was adjusting.

12

Reflections
and Hopes

I think often about what a sedate person I have become, involuntarily, since the onset of lupus. I used to keep a very energetic pace, and valued my independence tremendously. Now there are many things I simply cannot do. It is almost like having two lives, and I look back on my "first life" with envy and sadness.

Most noticeable to an outside observer are the changes in my activities. Reading and playing board games with the girls have replaced shopping, biking, and taking long walks. I no longer entertain large groups of family and friends, or stay up late. I miss dancing with Eddie and playing racquetball with my friends. I long to hold my nephews and nieces, and my friends' babies, but my muscles won't allow it. As the "simple pleasures" become memories, I realize how much I used to take all of this for granted.

Even more difficult to accept are the changes that only I see. There is a fearful part of me that never existed before. The part that has become proficient at covering up severe pain can't hide the pain from *me*. I worry about how much my body can endure and for how long.

These fears intensify when I realize that at 40 I am old beyond my years, with a body that does not have the stamina to keep up with senior citizens. I worry about being here to see major events in my children's lives, as I recall a special friend of mine with lupus, who died at a very young age. I cringe to see frail, balding chemotherapy patients, as my own fears of the long-term effects of treatment surface.

These thoughts are uncomfortable for me to reflect on even in these pages, and I try not to dwell on them. Yet, the fears rise up in me regularly, and they are unnerving.

Having lupus has also resulted in dramatic role changes in our home, and underlying resentment. This is an area any chronically ill person needs to be very honest about. Because the disease came on so strong from the start, none of us was ready when our secure world turned upside down. My role as a wife and mother was challenged beyond my imagination. This certainly burst the "happy ever after" bubble which had encased our marriage. Eddie and I had assumed, as most of us do, that we were invulnerable to ill-health.

One of my biggest difficulties was lowering my perfectionistic standards. I had to erase all the "shoulds" that I had associated with the roles of wife and mother, which involved both my sense of obligation and my strong sense of pride. I learned that my children could walk to the bus stop in the rain, my husband could find the energy after a day of work to prepare dinner, store-bought cakes were just as special as ones I spent hours on. Eddie and the girls went places without me and had a good time. Family members celebrated holidays which I used to host, and did just as good a job. I learned that I could add the word "no" to my vocabulary, and that naps in the middle of the day were acceptable for adults. Most difficult to learn was that a mommy could be sick.

Undoubtedly, the first year was the worst. When I went from being active and involved to nearly immobile, *no* one liked it! The kids were upset, though they tried not to show it, that I was no longer available to take them to the lake, entertain their friends, run out on an impromptu shopping trip. For Eddie, it meant handling more and more household responsibility on less and less sleep. I felt terrible guilt at the recognition of what my condition was doing to each of them. Underlying all of this was the very reasonable fear that I would only become more disabled, or actually die.

Another problem was dealing with my family's denial of the disease, which only made it harder for me to accept. It is a popular belief, but a completely misleading one in the case of chronic illness, that anyone who is sick can go to a doctor and be made well. No one expects that you will continue to be ill and have to learn to live with your disease. The girls looked constantly to me to prove that I was getting better. Though it was clear to me that their expectations were motivated by fear, I continually fell short in their eyes.

This attitude of denial and fear was also clear in my extended family and among my friends, with a few exceptions. I just wasn't the same woman they knew, who stayed up partying, playing cards, entertaining. I sensed that they missed me, but I wasn't perceptive enough at the time to recognize their vulnerability, too. Close friends, even my very best friends, would let months go by without the slightest inquiry as to how I was doing. This was incomprehensible to me. Now I see how terribly frightening it must have been to have a good friend, about your own age and in your kind of family situation, just stop walking overnight. If a dozen doctors couldn't help, what could you hope to do? And the real fear: could the same tragedy happen to you? As I began to see through their eyes, I understood that I might not have been any more brave if I'd been in their position.

The fifteen months that I spent searching for a diagnosis were filled with pain, frustration, and humiliation. I saw dozens of physicians and underwent numerous hospitalizations, uncomfortable procedures, and repeat surgeries. I was placed in the position of having to justify my own illness and to question the authority and knowledge of the medical profession. I only persevered in my pursuit for an accurate diagnosis and effective treatment program because of the severity of my symptoms. Though I was constantly stymied, I had no choice.

It is an injustice to place anyone in a position in which, in addition to trying to cope with a debilitating illness, he or she has to utilize already depleted resources trying to convince the doctors that something is genuinely wrong. The longer this situation went on, the greater my need became to make my story known. I am concerned as I speculate about the number of other patients currently experiencing severe problems, while being told that their symptoms do not fall into any identifiable category.

I should note that it was clearly to my disadvantage that my blood tests were negative for lupus for so long. I have been told that I am in the minority on this count, and that most patients exhibiting the other symptoms of lupus—joint and muscle pain, facial rashes, hair loss, Raynaud's phenomenon—also show evidence of the disease in their bloodwork. It took a much more invasive procedure, the muscle biopsy, to confirm my diagnosis.

I hope that my story—which is a *common* one, as I've discovered—will encourage the medical community to ensure that diseases such as lupus are diagnosed much earlier and treated effectively at a less advanced stage. I urge patients in similar situations to continue looking for an answer. Do not give up until you are satisfied. Seek second and third opinions if you feel that you are making no progress or are not being taken seriously.

I also hope that my case discourages premature "psychosomatic" diagnoses. A disease can run rampant in a person long before measurable evidence surfaces. That person desperately needs medical attention *and respect* during the painful waiting period.

I know from talking with other chronically ill persons that many of the struggles I've encountered are not unique to me or to lupus patients. Living with a serious illness for which there is as yet no cure demands effective and continual coping skills. My advice is to make the most of your life, and I recommend the following things in particular:

1. Join a support group—if none exists in your area, start one. It is an enormous source of hope to know that you are not alone and that your experience can be helpful to others.

2. Learn all you can about your illness; educate yourself so you can act as an up-to-date resource.

3. Look into individual or group therapy, visualization, relaxation tapes—whatever works to keep you emotionally healthy.

4. Promote public awareness of difficult-to-diagnose illnesses. Write an article for your local paper. Offer to speak, by phone if necessary, with newly diagnosed patients at a nearby hospital. Start a letter campaign for increased research, or plan a fundraising event.

For the spouses of chronically ill persons, Eddie's advice is to teach yourself how to live day to day, rather than agonizing over an uncertain future. Try to be flexible—you don't know how your spouse will be feeling from one hour to the next on some days. Understand that plans may need to change abruptly. His most important suggestion is to keep your lines of communication clear and open, because the disease and its limitations demand it.

Most of all, remember that there is hope. Instead of asking "why me," ask yourself what you still have in your life that holds value for you, and what you can draw from your situation to make it positive. You may not have control over the *fact* of your disease, but you can control the quality of your response to it. Your thoughtful, positive response will—I know from experience—make it easier to live with your disease. And your efforts to stop this long and frightening wait for a diagnosis may make all the difference for those who come after us.

APPENDIX I

Lupus: An Overview, References and Resources

Written with Meg Cohen

WHAT IS LUPUS?

Systemic lupus erythematosus (SLE) is an autoimmune disease that can affect virtually any organ in the body, including the heart, brain, kidneys, lungs, joints, skin, and circulatory system. Lupus is characterized by a malfunction of the immune system's cells. The immune system, which is essential for protecting the body from infection, normally produces antibodies which fight off invading foreign cells or substances. However, people with lupus generate an unusually high amount of abnormal antibodies, and instead of fighting off infection, these antibodies begin to attack healthy tissue. In a sense, the body becomes allergic to itself. Inflammation often occurs in the areas where the antibody attacks take place.

Tissue damage can occur in two ways: Antibodies can attack and damage tissue directly, or damage can occur by inflammatory reaction. When antibodies in the blood mix with the material that they are fighting, an immune structure is formed. Usually the body is able to eliminate this substance, but in individuals with lupus, the immune structure can become trapped, causing an inflammatory reaction. Inflammation, caused by antibodies attacking healthy tissue, occurs in the body's connective or vascular tissue. Connective tissue is composed of collagen (a protein substance), fiber, and other supporting tissues, and links the cells and tissues of the body. Since connective tissue is located in all organs and systems, lupus can affect any part of the body.

WHO IS AFFECTED?

More than 500,000 people have lupus in the United States today, with approximately 16,000 new cases diagnosed each year.

A remarkably disproportionate number of young women are affected by the disease. Among children, lupus occurs three times as often in girls as in boys, while 90 to 95 percent of lupus patients between the ages of 13 and 40 are female.

The onset of lupus can and does occur at any age. The numbers of men and women with lupus are much more equal in the over-40 age group.

Lupus can affect all racial and ethnic groups. The disease has been most thoroughly studied in North America, where it is approximately three times more common among blacks as among Caucasians.

IS LUPUS HEREDITARY?

There is no conclusive evidence that lupus is hereditary, but it appears that a tendency towards developing lupus may be inherited. If a family member has lupus, the *possibility* of developing lupus increases. Research suggests that a combination of genetic factors, the presence of various sex hormones, and even environmental variables may affect an individual's chances of contracting lupus. Only about four percent of the children of individuals with lupus develop lupus themselves.

IS LUPUS CONTAGIOUS?

There has never been a recorded case of anyone catching lupus from another person. There is interest now in the possibility that environmental factors may set off the production of abnormal antibodies in family or household members of an SLE patient who are not related to the patient genetically. But there is no evidence that these environmental factors, on their own, can "cause" lupus.

IS LUPUS FATAL?

While lupus is a chronic illness with no known cure, the belief that lupus is always fatal is a misconception. Lupus can last a lifetime, but it is not necessarily progressive. Through medical advances and improved treatment plans, the likelihood of lupus being terminal has been greatly reduced. Of every 100 patients with lupus, ten or fewer may die of the disease. These deaths occur, for the most part, when lupus damages the major internal organs.

TWO TYPES OF LUPUS

Two main types of lupus exist: discoid lupus and systemic lupus. While both can follow the flare-up/remission pattern (discussed in the next section), discoid is considered a much milder form and poses no real threat to health.

DISCOID LUPUS: Discoid or "cutaneous" lupus affects the skin. No other systems are involved, and there is no evidence of internal symptoms. It can be painful and may result in scarring.

Discoid lupus is characterized by patchy disc-shaped lesions which usually appear on the scalp, face, neck, and upper part of the chest. Lesions often assume the classic "butterfly" pattern, extending over the bridge of the nose and onto the cheeks. If attended to promptly, lesions may clear up quickly, without scarring.

Persons with discoid lupus must avoid direct sunlight and follow a carefully monitored medication plan. Approximately five percent of patients with discoid lupus develop systemic lupus.

SYSTEMIC LUPUS: Systemic lupus can attack any part of the body. It affects the internal organs, and its severity depends on which organs are affected and to what extent. Systemic lupus may include skin rashes, but it is the other internal symptoms that clearly distinguish it from discoid lupus.

Every case of lupus is unique. Individuals with lupus have different combinations of symptoms and may experience these symptoms in different ways. In general, people with systemic lupus suffer most from low-grade fevers, fatigue, occasional rashes, and joint pain or swelling.

WHAT ARE THE SYMPTOMS?

The most common symptoms of lupus are weakness

and fatigue, low-grade fevers, and all-over body aching. Symptoms tend to flare and subside mysteriously, with no warning. Flare-ups can be controlled by medication, and sometimes symptoms disappear completely, resulting in a state of remission from the disease which may be sustained for months or even years.

SKIN: Rashes (e.g., the butterfly facial rash), lesions, ulcers, or inflammation may occur. Rashes due to sun exposure occur in about 40 percent of lupus patients. Skin tends to bruise more easily and more frequently. Hair loss is common, as is Raynaud's phenomenon, in which the skin of the fingers and toes turns white or bluish from lack of circulation.

CHEST: Individuals with lupus may experience chest pain as a result of inflammation of the membranes surrounding the lungs or heart. Difficulty in breathing, shortness of breath, or a rapid heart beat may result. Chest pain may also be caused by inflammation in the rib and abdominal areas.

JOINTS: Joint pain is extremely common among lupus patients. This arthritis is characterized by swelling, redness, and stiffness, and may affect one or several joints.

BLOOD: Lupus patients have been known to have low red blood cell counts (anemia) as well as decreases in white blood cells (increasing their susceptibility to infection). However, if infection is already trapped in the body, the white blood cell count may increase significantly. Lupus patients may also have a false positive result for syphilis.

DIGESTIVE SYSTEM: Evidence that the digestive tract is involved may include stomach pain, cramps, nausea, vomiting, diarrhea, or constipation.

KIDNEYS: The possibility of kidney disease is one of the most serious aspects of lupus. Since no pain is associated with the early stages of a kidney disorder, a physician should be consulted regularly to test for any kidney dysfunction.

NERVOUS SYSTEM: Patients with nervous system involvement may experience headaches, seizures, temporary paralysis, or episodes of psychotic behavior.

The fact that a patient has abnormalities in several different organs or systems is often a doctor's best clue that he or she may be dealing with lupus. Remember, the general symptoms are experienced by the majority of persons with lupus, and while some people have *some* of the other symptoms, most people have only a few.

HOW IS LUPUS DIAGNOSED?

The diagnostic process is long and painstaking. It has been suggested that it takes an average of eight years for a person to be conclusively diagnosed with lupus! However, as mentioned above, lupus should be suspected in any individual with a multisystem disease accompanied by joint pain.

A critical part of diagnosing lupus is thorough testing of the immune system. Some of the best diagnostic tools are the anti-nuclear antibody test (ANA), the anti-DNA antibody test, and the anti-Sm antibody (a nuclear antibody named after a lupus patient) test. Doctors also check for the presence of immune complexes and a low serum complement level.

There are many reasons why lupus is difficult to

diagnose. It presents itself in countless variations. Each lupus patient has a different combination of symptoms and different complaints. Misdiagnoses are common, as physicians may believe that a person's symptoms are caused by some other better-known illness. Doctors must eliminate a large number of diseases which lupus mimics before they can offer a confident diagnosis.

Also, symptoms may come and go, or seem random and difficult to describe. Even the patient can become confused as to just how sick he or she really is. It may seem foolish to complain of feeling "heavy" or "tired all the time," so the person hesitates to seek medical attention.

Finally, laboratory tests are not always accurate, and may show a false positive or false negative result. A person can be very ill for months or years before definitive evidence of lupus appears in their bloodwork.

THE ELEVEN CRITERIA: Eleven criteria have been established for the purpose of diagnosing patients with lupus.* Physicians require that four of the 11 criteria be met in order to make a positive diagnosis of lupus. However, a tentative diagnosis can be made with fewer criteria. Lupus should be suspected if any criterion in the list is present and unexplained, particularly in a woman between the ages of 13 and 40.

1. Malar rash: Facial redness, or a rash on the cheekbone area.

2. Discoid rash: Red, raised patches and sometimes scaling. Healed lesions may appear as scars.

---

*   Revised criteria published by the American Rheumatism Association, 1982.

3. Photosensitivity: Extreme reaction to sunlight, even with minimal exposure.

4. Oral ulcers: Frequent occurrence of ulcers in the mouth, nose, or throat.

5. Arthritis: Non-erosive arthritis (not accompanied by any marked deformity) characterized by tenderness and swelling, although joint pain can occur without swelling. Must occur in two or more joints, which may include feet, ankles, knees, hips, fingers, wrists, elbows, shoulders, and lower jaw.

6. Pleurisy or pericarditis: Pleurisy is the inflammation of the sac surrounding the lungs. Its symptoms are chest pain with breathing and/or breathlessness. Pericarditis is an inflammation of the membranes that surround the heart. This condition often results in severe chest pain.

7. Kidney disorder: There are two types of kidney disease. Proteinuria is the existence of excessive protein in the urine. The second type involves "blood cell casts," the presence of abnormal antibodies in the urine. Kidney disorders are not detectable until in their advanced stages.

8. Neurologic disorder: Seizures (convulsions) or psychotic behavior occurring without the use of drugs or an obvious metabolic problem.

9. Blood disorder: One possible problem is hemolytic anemia, the spontaneous breakdown of red blood cells. However, this is a common disorder and not specific to lupus patients. A

second possible problem is leukopenia, a low white blood count. Individuals with lupus often have a low white count, and since the job of white blood cells is to fight off infection, the existence of leukopenia is significant in the diagnosis of lupus. A third potential blood problem is lymphopenia, a decrease in the number of lymphocytes—a type of white blood cell. A fourth problem is thrombocytopenia, which involves the number of platelets in the blood and may result in abnormal bleeding.

10. Immunologic disorder: LE cells are discovered in approximately 60 percent of all individuals who have lupus, and are rarely found in people without lupus. Laboratory tests should show the presence of two or more LE cells on any particular occasion. People with lupus also often demonstrate a false positive reaction to the test for syphilis. The syphilis test is important diagnostically because physicians are able to distinguish between a positive reaction due to abnormal lupus antibodies and real syphilis.

11. Antinuclear antibodies: A positive test for the production of antinuclear antibodies (ANA). The ANA test was designed for the purpose of detecting lupus. A positive ANA test is often essential to the diagnostic process.

The above criteria can exist in isolation as well as in any combination. However, with the exception of the butterfly rash and the ANA test, none of the criteria is specific to lupus. The combination of the criteria and the duration and severity of the manifestations is what determines whether or not a person has lupus.

HOW IS LUPUS TREATED?

Since each case of lupus is unique, physicians must design a special treatment program for each patient. The patient's treatment plan must be closely monitored, and the lines of communication should be open and honest. Because there is no known cure for lupus, treatment is symptomatic and aimed at the suppression of flare-ups in order to reduce the debilitating impact on the patient. It is important to note that at this stage of our knowledge about lupus, suppressing the symptoms is the same thing as suppressing the disease. Ideally, medication may result in a state of remission during which the symptoms are no longer present.

Aspirin, ibuprofen, and a number of prescription medications known as Non-Steroidal Anti-Inflammatory Drugs (NSAIDS) are used to reduce inflammation and thus tissue damage.

Steroids are the most common drug prescribed for the treatment of severe cases of lupus. If steroids are unsuccessful in suppressing symptoms, and a patient is severely ill, a physician may administer immunosuppressant drugs. Immunosuppressants are still considered investigational, and, like steroids, are potentially dangerous. Both of these classes of drugs can have very serious side effects, which patients should be aware of before beginning treatment.

The patient plays the central role in his/her treatment. Although physicians can offer medical advice, medication, and expertise, and family and friends can lend crucial emotional support, only the patient can make the everyday decisions that affect the quality of his/her life. It is important to learn ways to keep stress to a minimum. Exercise and good nutrition are factors which the patient can control. The medical facts about lupus are important, but equally critical to successful management of the disease is faithful attention to one's own social and emotional life.

REFERENCES

Ronald I. Carr, M.D. *Lupus Erythematosus: A Handbook for Physicians, Patients, and Their Families.* St. Louis: Lupus Foundation of America, 1986.

Terri Nass. *Lupus Erythematosus: Handbook for Nurses.* Lupus Society of Wisconsin, P. O. Box 16621, Milwaukee, WI 53216, 1985. (The author is both a nurse and a lupus patient.)

Robert H. Phillips, M.D. *Coping with Lupus.* Wayne, NJ: Avery Publishing Group, 1984.

Sefra Kobrin Pitzele. *We Are Not Alone: Learning to Live with Chronic Illness.* Minneapolis: Thompson and Co., Inc., 1985.

Steven J. Schostal. *Lupus Patients in Relation to Family and Friends.* Greater Atlanta Chapter of Lupus Foundation of America, 2814 New Spring Road, Atlanta, GA 30339.

RESOURCES

American Lupus Society
23751 Madison Street
Torrance, CA 90505
(213) 373-1335

Lupus Erythematosus Support Club
8039 Nova Court
North Charleston, SC 29420

Lupus Foundation of America
1717 Massachusetts Avenue, Suite 203
Washington, DC 20036
(800) 558-0121

Lupus Network
230 Ranch Drive
Bridgeport, CT 06606
(203) 372-5795

Check your phone book for a local chapter near you. The Lupus Foundation of America, for example, currently lists more than 100 chapters across the country.

Because of her concern for other lupus patients, the author welcomes their correspondence and will make every effort to answer each letter personally. She may be reached through the publisher:

Eileen Radziunas
c/o Hunter House Inc., Publishers
P.O. Box 847
Claremont, CA 91711

Appendix *II*

Other "Imposter Diseases"

Written with Meg Cohen

Lupus is only one of many illnesses with unknown causes and as yet unknown cures. The term "imposter disease" refers to a diverse group of illnesses which share the following features:

— Symptoms which mimic other diseases. As was seen so clearly in this narrative, well-informed doctors may arrive at completely different diagnoses because the patient's symptoms are non-specific, or can be associated with a disease with which the doctor is more familiar.

— A variable presentation of symptoms. An imposter disease usually presents itself in the "flare-up/remission" pattern, so that both the patient and the doctor become confused by symptoms that come and go or vary greatly in their severity. Also, patients with the same disease have quite different symptoms. For instance, while oral ulcers are included in the eleven criteria for diagnosing lupus, not all lupus patients develop this symptom. The symptoms appear in many different combinations.

— Symptoms that are not detectable through standard medical exams and tests. Imposter diseases generally do not have any one test that can identify them conclusively. Thus, the physician needs to be watching for a suspicious combination of problems, rather than a particular outcome on any given test.

The diagnostic process for imposter diseases is long, exhausting, costly, and often painful. Both patient and doctor become distressed by misleading symptoms and test results. The extended diagnostic period can tax the patient's physical, psychological, and interpersonal well-being. Because imposter diseases often induce psychoneurotic symptoms, patients are frequently labeled hypochondriacs or neurotics and referred to the care of a psychiatrist. Before being correctly diagnosed, many patients endure depression, numerous misdiagnoses and thus mistreatment, and sometimes the breakup of a marriage or important friendships because of the constant strain.

It is clear that physicians are not wholly to blame for this traumatic process. The mysterious nature of imposter diseases makes them extremely tricky to diagnose. Doctors for the most part would rather be quite certain about a diagnosis, even if it takes repeated testing and second and third opinions, than to misdiagnose and consequently mistreat what is obviously a serious illness.

Multiple sclerosis, Epstein-Barr virus, temporomandibular joint (TMJ) syndrome, candidiasis, and endometriosis can all be considered imposter diseases. (The list could be made longer to include, for example, thyroid disorders, myasthenia gravis, premenstrual syndrome, and the group of diseases now being called "environmental illnesses.") Although they vary greatly, these illnesses all present deceiving symptoms and are to some extent difficult to diagnose. The majority of these diseases affect more women than men; some are specific to women.

MULTIPLE SCLEROSIS

Multiple sclerosis (MS) is a disease of the central nervous system. It affects scattered areas of the brain and spinal cord and interferes with the brain's ability to control such basic functions as sight, coordination, and speech. MS is the most common nervous system disease among young adults in the United States. Although cases do occur in children under age 10 and in adults over 60, MS is most likely to strike in the intermediate years. At present, MS is not preventable or curable.

Multiple sclerosis disrupts communication between the central nervous system and the other parts of the body. Healthy nerve fibers are insulated by myelin, a fatty material which aids in the flow of signals. In MS patients, the myelin breaks down and is replace by scar tissue (sclera), which blocks and distorts the flow of messages. The messages from the brain either never reach their intended sites, or they arrive jumbled, and thus basic bodily functions become uncontrollable.

Although there is currently no way to determine who will contract MS, scientists have developed several theories about its origins.

1. Viral attack: When a virus enters the body, it

multiplies rapidly inside the cells. Viruses usually create obvious symptoms quickly, but certain slow-acting viruses tend to appear and reappear, sometimes causing different symptoms each time they surface. Some slow-acting viruses incubate inside the body for months or even years before creating any signs of illness. MS may be caused by a slow-acting virus or a delayed reaction to a common virus.

2. Immune reaction: MS, like lupus, may be caused by an autoimmune reaction. The body's immune system may begin to attack its own myelin-producing cells instead of destroying invading viruses and bacteria.

3. A combination of these two factors: Because viruses invade and take over body cells, the immune system may become confused and attack both the body's healthy cells and the invading virus.

Since the cause of MS is so uncertain, it is difficult to accurately predict who is at risk. However, there is a pattern. Symptoms usually appear between the ages of 17 and 40; the illness seldom strikes people under 15 or over 50. Also more women than men develop MS, at a ratio of 3 to 2.

Studies suggest that environmental factors play a role in the development of MS. People who spend the first 15 years of life in areas between 40 and 60 degrees north and south of the equator have less of a chance of developing the disease than do those who spend this period farther away from the equator. People in areas with high standards of sanitation are also more susceptible to MS, possibly because they are not exposed to some factor that would help build immunity to the disease.

MS is not contagious or hereditary. However, susceptibility to autoimmune diseases appears to be at least partially genetic, so even though MS itself is not hereditary, a hereditary factor may be at work which makes the individual more likely to develop this type of disease.

The symptoms of MS vary greatly, both from person to person and from time to time in the same person. General symptoms include: seeing double, or uncontrolled eye movements; partial or complete paralysis of any part of the body; shaking of the hands; loss of bladder or bowel control; problems with speech, such as slurring; staggering or loss of balance; weakness and fatigue; numbness or a pricking feeling; loss of coordination; an obvious dragging of the feet.

MS patients rarely have all of these symptoms. Early symptoms are usually slight and disappear without treatment. As the disease progresses, symptoms may return, increase in number, or become more severe. Symptoms also vary depending on which part of the nervous system is affected. For example, MS occurring in the spinal cord may result in weakness, numbness, and paralysis of the arms and legs.

As with lupus, none of these symptoms is specific to MS, and could signify the presence of some other disease. The early symptoms are often so slight that they hardly warrant medical attention. There is no laboratory test available to conclusively determine the presence of MS, but two basic criteria are used in diagnosing the disease. The first is numbness or tingling of the hands and feet, along with unexplained weakness or paralysis. (Two or more parts of the central nervous system must be involved.) The second criterion is the flare-up/remission pattern of symptoms appearing and disappearing without warning. This is not typical of other nervous system diseases. A person diagnosed with MS should not despair. Most MS patients lead long, active lives, and the disease can be minimized with proper management. MS patients must eat properly, stay well rested, and attend to infections promptly. Physical therapy is also important. Medication is sometimes prescribed to relieve specific symptoms, for example, muscle relaxants for spasms. More severe cases may require stronger medication. Since the course of MS is unpredictable, continuous medical supervision is essential. There are also excellent support groups, research centers, information services, and publications available.

EPSTEIN-BARR VIRUS

The Epstein-Barr virus (EBV) is a rare, severe illness that involves the major organs. EBV is typically accompanied by such serious conditions as chronic hepatitis, pneumonia, and anemia. It is usually transmitted through saliva; however, it can also be spread through blood transfusions. Symptoms include fever, rashes, hair loss, swollen glands, and joint and muscle pain. EBV, like MS, affects twice as many women as men.

EBV attacks the B cells, one type of white blood cell in the body's immune system. The virus enters the B cells and releases its own genetic material. It quickly multiplies and begins to damage the normal, healthy cells.

Epstein-Barr is actually a very common virus; almost everyone is chronically infected with it by early adulthood. EBV is thought responsible for a wide variety of diseases throughout the world, rang-ing from the benign to the fatal. Two of the more severe illnesses linked to EBV are Burkitt's lymphoma and nasopharyngeal carcinoma, both forms of cancer. Mononucleosis is the most common benign infection associated with EBV, which also seems to play a part in the development of chronic fatigue syndrome (CFS), though it is not the primary infectious agent in CFS, and the two illnesses are sometimes confused.

Within the first few months of initial infection, most EBV patients "shed" the disease. This means that the virus is active and is being discharged in the saliva, which may increase the likelihood of transmission. It is possible to be infected with EBV by a healthy person who is shedding the infection, or by a person with an obvious illness, such as mononucleosis. EBV is, however, relatively difficult to transmit.

Epstein-Barr is a member of the herpes family of viruses. As with all forms of herpes, once a person is infected with the disease, he or she remains infected for life. The body naturally develops an immunity against further outbreaks of the disease associated with the virus, but the virus is still present in the body, in a latent state. Some people's immunity may not be strong enough to prevent symptomatic recurrences.

There is a test for detecting the Epstein-Barr virus. The EBV serology test measures the presence of antibodies to the virus, from which the actual presence of the virus can be inferred. However, EBV tests are not completely reliable, and many healthy individuals produce abnormal test results.

TEMPOROMANDIBULAR JOINT SYNDROME

Temporomandibular joint syndrome (TMJ) is a pain syndrome that can lead to any of the following symptoms: headaches; aching or stiff neck or shoulders; backaches; ringing or pain in the ears; popping, clicking, or pain in the jaw joint; facial pain; numbness in the fingers and toes; dizziness; and tooth pain.

These symptoms are caused by muscle spasms in the head, neck, shoulders, and back—the muscles that control the lower jaw—but the spasms actually originate in a gearing conflict in the teeth. The severity of symptoms varies from patient to patient, and the source of the problem is difficult to determine because it does not affect the appearance of the teeth or even appear to be related to that area of the body.

The most common way for a muscle to rebel when under strain is to go into spasm, which results in a painful contraction of the muscle. When a muscle goes into spasm, it sends a message back to the central nervous system, which, in turn, interprets the signal and causes the muscle to contract even more. A painful cycle begins. Because the muscles for chewing (the mastication muscles) are in the head, spasms may result in headaches. A headache is the most common symptom of TMJ, and it is usually the severity of the headache that drives a person to the doctor's office.

Because TMJ is a disorder related to muscle spasm, standard lab tests yield no information toward a correct diagnosis. Definite clinical signs of TMJ are seldom seen, so physicians are wholly dependent on the description of symptoms provided by the patient.

The temporomandibular joint is one of the most important yet poorly understood joints in the body. Extensive research on TMJ has only been undertaken in the last 25 years. Because of its unique anatomic position and association with other structures, dentists often consider it outside their realm of responsibility and treatment. The symptoms of TMJ cross over the medical and dental disciplinary lines, leaving a discrepancy as to who's in charge.

It remains a mystery why some people are more susceptible to muscle spasms than others, but it appears to have much to do with the relationship between an individual's pain threshold and stress level. The potential for TMJ problems exists in almost everyone—80 to 90 percent of the population has a tooth-gearing discrepancy. The absence of many of the major symptoms of TMJ in the majority of people with the disorder is a tribute to the neuromuscular system's ability to protect itself. However, this ability also masks the problem and makes it difficult to reach a diagnosis.

The majority of TMJ patients are between the ages of 30 and 50 and, again, more women are diagnosed with the illness than men. It is triggered by trauma or stress. Trauma can take the form of whiplash, a sports injury, a blow to the head or face, etc. Stress, on the other hand, must be related to the existence of a tooth-gearing problem in order to produce TMJ.

A proper diagnosis is the key to successful treatment, which may include:

1. Medication: Controlled, monitored medication is essential in the early stages. Muscle relaxants, nonsteroidal anti-inflammatory drugs, and mild narcotics such as codeine are used to subdue the pain. Drugs should be used to assist the diagnostic process, not as primary agents or long-term treatment. A short duration is usually prescribed; a week on any of these medications may be considered enough.

2. Occlusal intervention: The most common method is the creation and use of an acrylic splint. The splint is designed specifically for the patient's particular problem, and placed over the teeth to correct the misalignment.

3. Physical therapy: Exercises designed especially for the patient's problem. It is important that the patient not over-exercise, because strain may cause more muscle fatigue and pain.

4. Surgical intervention: Surgery is only used as a last resort because of its questionable success rate.

The first two areas of treatment are designed to break the cycle of muscle spasm and relieve pain. By artificially achieving the proper relationship between the upper and lower jaw, the lower jaw is allowed to move freely again. When active treatment is complete, most patients are cured of TMJ.

CANDIDIASIS

Candidiasis is the general term for a yeast infection caused by the colonization of the Candida species. Its most common cause is *candida albicans*, a class of fungus present in everyone's body, which usually inhabits the mouth, esophagus, intestines, vagina, and skin. Unlike most other types of fungi, *candida albicans* is transmissible. The most frequent manifestations of candidiasis are superficial lesions, especially in or around the mouth or vagina. Symptoms of candidiasis include lethargy, cystitis, vaginitis, emotional explosiveness (often uncontrollable crying), and decreased libido.

Yeasts are single-celled organisms belonging to

the fungus kingdom. As long as the immune system keeps its balance, the presence of yeast in the body does not cause problems; a healthy immune system can prevent an overgrowth of yeast. However, certain factors affecting the body's chemistry can drastically upset the immune system's balance. Pregnancy, oral contraceptive use, and treatment with antibiotics are a few of these. Antibiotics kill healthy intestinal bacteria, which allows yeast to flourish and increases the movement of yeast to all areas of the body. Immunosuppressant drugs weaken the immune system. As yeast colonies multiply, they release a variety of yeast toxins into the bloodstream. The immune system initially attempts to produce antibodies to counter these toxins, but it eventually goes into a frenzy, becomes weakened, and either cannot fight off substances that a healthy system would have no problem with, or begins to make antibodies to substances that are not enemies.

There are several steps you can follow to avoid the growth of yeast:

1. Reduce the exposure to yeast foods in your diet.

2. Begin a low-carbohydrate diet. Yeast colonies cannot live and reproduce efficiently on fats and proteins alone, so by depriving them of high levels of carbohydrates, you help kill them off.

3. Avoid antibiotics unless absolutely necessary.

4. If possible, avoid contraceptive hormones.

5. Minimize your exposure to high-mold environments.

Anti-yeast prescription drugs are available to

reduce the existence of candida colonies in the body. The use of these should be carefully monitored by a physician. Also, it is important for people with candida infections to strengthen their immune systems by eating a nutritious diet, avoiding immunosuppressant medication, keeping their stress level low, and taking candida extract (under a physician's care), which also helps to relieve painful symptoms.

Although candidiasis can present itself as an obvious yeast infection, some individuals suffer from candida infections without displaying any overt symptoms. Because of the frequent absence of visible symptoms, candidiasis can be difficult to diagnose. It is often dismissed as a psychosomatic illness, and, in its milder forms, may be considered simply a nuisance. It is important to remember that a candida infection that goes undetected or untreated can cause more serious immune system problems down the line.

ENDOMETRIOSIS

Endometriosis is an enigmatic and often extremely painful disease. Endometrial cells are normally found only in the lining of the uterus. In endometriosis, these cells are found in and surrounding other organs of the female reproductive system, the bladder, intestines, or even in such unexpected places as the lungs or head. The endometrial cells continue to function in these other parts of the body as though they were still in the uterus. That is, they build up with the menstrual cycle, bleed, and attempt to slough off. Because there is no place for them to go, they can cause internal bleeding, cysts, and swelling.

Endometriosis is associated with miscarriage, ectopic pregnancy, ruptured ovarian cysts, and infertility. Fifteen to 25 percent of infertile women are diagnosed with endometriosis. Estimates of the number of women with the disease who are infertile range from 20 percent to a remarkable 66 percent.

The cause of endometriosis is not known. There are several major theories concerning this misplacement of cells. The direct implantation theory suggests that the cells are planted in the pelvic cavity by the menstrual flow backing up through the fallopian tubes. The celomic metaplasia theory postulates the existence in the body, from birth, of "multipotential" cells which can develop into endometrial cells. The vascular dissemination theory suggests that endometrial cells enter the uterine vasculature or the lymphatic vessels at menstruation and are carried to distant sites along these channels. Although it is generally thought of as a single disease entity, endometriosis actually involves a wide array of clinical presentations, and there is some speculation that it may not be a disease at all, but rather a clinical manifestation of some more common, underlying illness.

Endometriosis affects approximately one to two percent of the general population. It often develops during adolescence, but is not usually recognized until later in life, typically between the ages of 25 and 45. Although it is not hereditary, an unaffected individual with an affected blood relative has a seven percent chance of developing endometriosis, as compared to a one percent chance for non-blood-related persons. If not relieved through hormonal treatment or surgery, the disease will progress with continued hormonal stimulation until menopause, when it usually recedes.

Some of the symptoms associated with endometriosis include pain and cramping with ovulation, menstruation, or during intercourse, signs or symptoms of urinary tract infection, extreme or irregular periods, and unusual abdominal masses. A seldom-recognized but relatively significant indication of the disease is spotting occurring three to seven days before the start of a period.

The problems most women have in obtaining a diagnosis are that the symptoms tend to come and go with menstruation, which doctors may dismiss as "normal," and that the range of severity of the symptoms is so wide. One woman with endometriosis may be in constant pain, while another only discovers that she has the disease when she goes in for infertility tests or has surgery for an unrelated problem. To date, physicians and researchers have not reached a clear understanding of the cause of endometriosis or its strong relationship to infertility.

REFERENCES

Mary Lou Ballweg. *Overcoming Endometriosis*. New York: Congdon and Weed, Inc., 1987.

The Boston Women's Health Book Collective. *The New Our Bodies, Ourselves*. New York: Simon and Schuster, 1984.

Constance DeSwaan and Niels H. Lauersen. *The Endometriosis Answer Book: New Hope, New Help*. New York: Rawson Associates, 1988.

"EBV 'Isn't an Agent of Chronic Fatigue Syndrome.'" *Internal Medicine News*, July 15-31, 1989, p. 17.

M. A. Epstein and B. C. Achong, eds. *The Epstein-Barr Virus: Recent Advances*. New York: John Wiley and Sons, Inc., 1986.

A. Richard Goldman, D.D.S., with Virginia McCullough. *TMJ Syndrome: The Overlooked Diagnosis*. New York: Simon and Schuster, Inc., 1987.

Bryan Matthews. *Multiple Sclerosis: The Facts.* 2nd edition. London: Oxford University Press, 1985.

F. C. Odds. *Candida and Candidiasis.* 2nd edition. London: Bailliere Tindall, 1988.

Julia Older. *A Woman's Guide to Endometriosis.* New York: Charles Scribner's Sons, Inc., 1984.

Randall T. Schapiro. *Symptom Management in Multiple Sclerosis.* New York: Demos Publications, Inc. 1987.

Emery A. Wilson, ed. *Endometriosis.* New York: Alan R. Liss, 1987.

RESOURCES

International Health Foundation (candidiasis)
P.O. Box 1000RH
Jackson, TN 38302

National CEBV Syndrome Association
P.O. Box 230108
Portland, OR
(503) 684-5261

National Multiple Sclerosis Society
205 East 42nd Street
New York, NY 10017
Toll-free: (800) 624-8236 or (800) 227-3166

U.S.-Canadian Endometriosis Association
P. O. Box 92187
Milwaukee, WI 53202
Toll-free: (800) 992-ENDO (in the U.S.)

ORDER FORM

NAME

ADDRESS

CITY/STATE   ZIP

POSTAL CODE   COUNTRY

TITLE	QTY	PRICE	TOTAL
The Enabler		@ $ 6.95	
Exclusively Female		@ $ 5.95	
Getting High in Natural Ways		@ $ 6.95	
Healthy Aging *(paperback)*		@ $ 11.95	
Healthy Aging *(hard cover)*		@ $ 17.95	
Lupus: My Search for a Diagnosis		@ $ 6.95	
Menopause Without Medicine		@ $ 11.95	
Nutrition and Your Body		@ $ 9.95	
Once A Month *4th Edition*		@ $ 9.95	
PMS: Premenstrual Syndrome		@ $ 6.95	

Shipping costs:
First book: $2.00
($3.00 for Canada)
Each additional book:
$.50 ($1.00 for Canada)
For UPS rates and bulk orders call us at
(714) 624-2277

TOTAL
Less discount @_____%   ( )
TOTAL COST OF BOOKS   _____
Calif. residents add sales tax   _____
Shipping & handling   _____
TOTAL ENCLOSED
Please pay in U.S. funds only

❏ Check   ❏ Money Order   ❏ Visa   ❏ M/C

Card # _____ Exp date _____

Signature _____

Phone number _____

Complete and mail to:
Hunter House Inc., Publishers
PO Box 847, Claremont, CA 91711
❏ Check here to receive our book catalog